FIX TIGHT

HIP FLEXORS

The Ultimate Cure to Reduce Joint Pain and Increase Muscle Flexibility

DAN MATTHEWS

TABLE OF CONTENTS

Hip flexors

The hip flexors help balance the back and the pelvic muscles. Three key muscles regularly become tight and abbreviated because of exercises undertaken in day by day living. These are the iliacus, psoas major, and the rectus femoris. The iliacus and the psoas major are regularly alluded to as the iliopsoas because they share a similar inclusion at the lesser trochanter of the femur. The psoas minor embeds on the prevalent ramus of the pubis bone and for the most part supports the normal lordotic ebb and flow of the spine, however, it is just found in about 40% of the population.

The psoas major starts on the foremost surface of the lumbar vertebrae and runs over the pubis bone and embeds into the lesser trochanter of the femur. This muscle flexes the hip, yet in addition, it affects the lordotic bend of the lumbar vertebrae. The rectus femoris has a proximal connection at the hip bone socket and inserts into the tibial tuberosity. This long muscle has a job in both hip flexion and leg extension.

At the point when these muscles are under steady strain due to ergonomics and constant postural situating, they may turn out to be tight and shortened. This can bring cause them to pull forward on the lumbar vertebrae, causing hyperlordosis and making the pelvis tilt anteriorly. This is regularly found in individuals who stay seated for a drawn-out period, for example, office laborers, software engineers, and other people who end up sitting at a work area for quite a long time each day.

It is essential to give training on legitimate ergonomics, development, and self-care to these people. Working in the pelvic area isn't simple for some counselors and customers. There are warnings and restrictions that should be addressed and talked through before being addressed to these muscles. There are passionate and comfortable viewpoints about working in the lower pelvic area.

A few customers see this region as excessively close to home or too private to permit the therapist's hands to go here. Different observations include the internal organs, for example, the digestive organs, uterus, kidneys, and bladder. As the iliacus and psoas travel under the inguinal ligament and insert into the lesser trochanter of the femur, there is also the femoral triangle, which should be worked around. Body positioning can be valuable to help get to these muscles in a less intrusive manner while ensuring the comfort of the customer.

The hip flexors can be found linking the highest point of the femur, which is the biggest bone in the body, to the lower back, hips, and crotch.

There are different hip flexor muscles that all work to enable an individual to be mobile.

They include:

- The iliacus and psoas significant muscles that are also referred to as the iliopsoas
- The rectus femoris, which is a part of an individual's quadriceps

Abuse or overstretching of these muscles and ligaments can bring about damage and cause pain and reduced mobility.

Symptoms of a hip flexor strain

Many individuals who experience hip flexor strain will also have these symptoms:

- Sudden, sharp pain in the hip or pelvis after an injury to the region
- A squeezing or holding sensation in the muscles of the upper leg region
- The upper leg feels delicate and sore
- Loss of strength in the front of the crotch along with a pulling sensation
- Muscle spasms in the hip or thighs
- Inability to keep kicking, jumping, or sprinting
- Reduced mobility and uneasiness while moving, including limping
- Discomfort and pain in the upper leg region, which feels constant
- Swelling or pain around the hip or thigh area
- Tightness or stiffness after being stationary, for example, after resting
- Constant impairing pain or uneasiness in the crotch or hip, in any event, when sitting
- Decreased scope of movement particularly recognizable when kicking, lunging, running, and bending
- Tenderness, swelling, and pain in the upper leg or crotch; the affected area may hurt when squeezed
- Muscle spasms or potentially spasms in the hip or thigh that are painful and impact growth
- Weakness in the groin area that may make certain exercises, for example, kicking, difficult or impossible
- Change in step, pain, the diminished scope of movement, and different factors influence walking

Hip flexor pain is ordinarily worse during specific exercises or specific developments, for example,

- Prolonged sitting, for example, sitting during the day for office work or a long vehicle trip
- Going up or down stairs
- Bending the knee to the chest (for instance, to tie a shoe)
- Bending over to get something
- Pushing off the affected leg to change direction while running or skating

An individual doesn't need to relate to these triggers to have hip flexor pain.

Hip flexor pain is frequently felt in the hip or crotch and is aggravated by specific developments, for example, kicking, rotating at high speeds, or moving the knee towards the chest. The hidden reason for hip flexor horrible pain may be:

1. Hip flexor strain or tear. A strain or tear refers to the damage caused to a muscle or ligament when it is stretched excessively far. Regularly, a hip flexor strain or tear happens when someone does something suddenly, for example, changing direction while running. Muscle tears are rated on a reviewing framework (gentle to extreme) dictated by the seriousness of pain, loss of movement, and shortcomings in the affected area.

2. Hip flexor tendinopathy. Ligaments are the stringy structures that connect muscle to bone. Hip flexor tendinopathy which incorporates both tendonitis and tendinosis might be brought about by intense damage, for example, from a fall or auto crash, or by damage, for example, from running, gymnastics, or soccer. Moreover, hip flexor

tendinopathy can happen with age as the ligaments normally lose flexibility.

3. Iliopsoas bursitis. Iliopsoas bursitis happens when a hip's iliopsoas bursa gets aggravated. The iliopsoas bursa is a small, liquid-filled sac situated between the front of the hip joint and the iliopsoas muscle. This damage is frequently found in high-impact sports, for example, soccer, skiing, or artful dance. Iliopsoas bursitis can likewise be brought about by arthritis.

4. Hip impingement. In most energetic adults, hip impingement is brought about by unusual bone development and may make someone experience hip pain, for the most part in the groin area, and a decline in the hip's range of movement. There are 3 unique sorts of hip impingement—cam, pincer, and consolidated. The kind of hip impingement is controlled by the area of unusual bone development.

5. Hip labral tear. The hip labrum is a ring of the strong, adaptable ligament that edges the external edge of the hip attachment (hip bone socket) and takes into account a critical range of movement. At the point when damaged, it might cause front hip or crotch pain that is regularly depicted as a deep, dull, ache. Pain from a labral tear can show up progressively after some time or all of a sudden. Labral tears are ordinarily found in people who play sports that include running, kicking, or turning.

6. Osteoarthritis. Hip osteoarthritis is a typical type of joint inflammation that happens when the defensive ligament in the hip joint wears out after some time. This ligament ordinarily decreases friction between the hip's ball and socket during joint development. Osteoarthritis may cause hip tenderness, stiffness, and a loss of flexibility.

7. Overuse. Hip flexor pain can show up with no definite underlying conditions or wounds. In these cases, the fundamental reason might be misuse. People who regularly play sports that include running, kicking, or turning, for example, soccer or football, may experience pain from misuse.

8. Pelvic obliquity (tilted pelvis). Restorative experts use the term pelvic obliquity to refer to a pelvis that is misaligned or tilted forward. Pelvic obliquity is related to labour (in ladies), sitting for long periods, lack of stretching, and poor posture. Pelvic obliquity may cause muscles in the hip or groin area to feel tight.

9. Avascular putrefaction (osteonecrosis). Rarely, hip flexor pain is brought about by avascular rot, a condition that happens when blood supply to a bone is altogether decreased or cut off. Hip pain from avascular rot is frequently felt in the main point of the groin, thigh, or buttocks and may develop gradually. Avascular rot is regularly brought about by trauma to the joint, for example, a crack or break, yet can also be from too much steroids or liquor use.

Functions of Healthy Hip Flexors

Regardless of whether you're an athlete or not, the condition of your hip flexors is significant. Any development, including twisting around or pulling your knees toward your chest includes this gathering of hip muscles. At the point when you lift a basket of laundry, hunch down to get something off a low rack at the market or choose to take the stairs up to your office rather than the lift, you're asking your hip flexors to work.

Essentially standing up also requires having great hip flexor quality. If your hips are incapable or tight, your posture suffers, and your lower spine is put under more stress than it's intended to take. Your knees can also end up taking on an exaggerated burden as your body endeavors to make up for stiffness somewhere else. These kinds of imbalance characteristics may cause damage now or raise the danger of joint degeneration if they cause joint inflammation as you age.

During exercises or sports, hip flexors help stimulate the hips and glutes, expanding the capability of exercises, for example, squats and deadlifts. You need versatility in your hips to keep up the great structure during these developments and to help speed and power in different sorts of exercises. If you need to jump higher, run faster or lift more weight, you can't disregard the great muscles in your hips.

Why Your Hip Flexors are Tight
The strong, adaptable hip muscles you were born with are intended to control your legs all through your whole life. When you were a child, it was anything but difficult to get around, ride your bicycle, bounce around, swim and for the most part be as lively as you needed without getting up toward the beginning of the day and feeling like somebody was taking a flame thrower to your hips. What went wrong?

Present-day inactive ways of life, particularly among leading office workers, are, to a great extent at fault for interminable hip flexor issues. Sitting for long periods of time at disables the hip flexor muscles and causes "adaptive shortening," a condition where the muscles start to get shorter due to being comparably positioned for a long time. Indeed, even lively individuals can experience the ill effects of adaptive shortening if their chosen games include flexion, for example,

- Running
- Cycling
- Soccer
- Martial arts
- High-intensity sprinting

Disparities between hips and hamstrings can also cause hip flexor issues. Neglecting to stretch after exercise or concentrating a lot on the backs of your legs without also doing hip flexor exercises leaves some hip muscles free, while others keep on freezing up from lack of movement.

How would you know whether you have to strengthen your hip flexors? Be watchful for at least one of these symptoms:

- Lower back pain
- Difficulty standing upright
- Tender or stiff muscles in the hip region
- Pain in the upper groin
- Dull pain advancing to progressively serious discomfort
- Chronic hip tightness
- Weak stomach muscles
- Anterior pelvic tilt
- Knee pain

Neglecting to address tight hip flexor muscles could mean you'll need a hip replacement later on. This is one reason why hip flexor stretches to keep up a full range of movement in your hips is so significant. Less stretching can prompt unhealthy joints and untimely wear that requires careful intercession.

Sometimes, your symptoms may show a further developed or more major issue. Iliopsoas tendinitis, in which hip flexor ligaments become aggravated, is one possibility that causes tenderness and "snapping" in the hip joints. The strain on the hip flexors can make the muscles tear, and this condition can run from minor to serious contingent upon the degree of the damage.

Unlocking Your Hip Flexors for Pain Relief and Better Performance
If you've decided your discomfort was brought about by stiffness in your hip flexors, don't stress. You do not have to suffer with shortened or feeble hip muscles forever. A couple of basic hip flexor stretches can help relieve stiff hips, increase range of movement and strengthen areas experiencing lack of movement.

To capitalize on these hip stretches:

- Make sure your muscles are warm before beginning
- Hold each position for at least 30 seconds
- Maintain an ordinary breathing example
- Stay in charge of your body
- Don't push the stretch to a point where it feels painful

Deep stretching should consistently be done after an exercise or as a different session. Doing comprehensive static stretching before exercise can build up your risk of injury. Stretch on a mat or other soft surface to protect your back and knees.

Make sure to talk with your primary care physician before beginning any new kind of exercise, including deep stretching, to decide the most suitable routine for your condition.

If your hip flexors are damaged, odds are you recognize what's causing it-a lot of SoulCycle or an too much sitting at your work area. Less clear? Here are some instructions to fix it.

Perhaps you've taken a stab at taking a walk and doing stretches after class, yet those presumably haven't helped ease the hurt obviously. That is because the issue isn't entirely your hip flexors-it is your glutes, says Allison Heffron, D.C., a chiropractor at restoration center Physio Logic in Brooklyn. And, you don't have to stretch, you have to strengthen them.

Have you ever felt a sharp pain coming from the front of your pelvis down to the very top of your thigh each time you lift your leg? That is what we call a sore hip flexor.

Quick anatomy lesson:
Your hip flexors are a group of muscles that attach your pelvis to your femur (the bone in your upper leg) and assist it with lifting and lowering (just as do each smaller scale development in the middle). The biggest of the hip flexor muscles are the psoas muscle, which wraps from the rear of your spine around over the front of your pelvis to the highest point of your femur, and the iliac muscle, which connects the top front of your pelvis straight down to identical ligaments on the femur from the psoas.

"Ordinarily, hip flexors freeze if they're overused as a reaction to something separate from being underused-for the most part your glutes," says Heffron. Because of sitting throughout the day and hurrying through your squats, your glutes are never taught to work appropriately. (We know-you truly feel like you're connecting with your glutes during these exercises, however, if your hip flexors are sore, that is a significant sign you're not.)

"It's as though your glutes are the power change to kill the hip flexors. At the point when you're working out or even simply walking, and you center on stimulating the glutes, it inhibits overuse of the hip flexors. This enables the hip flexors to rest and be less taxed while the glutes carry out the responsibility they are intended to do," says Heffron.

Think about your hip flexors as the muscles controlling the front portion of your leg, and your gluteal muscles (every one of the three max, medi, and minimum) as the ones controlling the back. When the two are ending and working in a state of harmony, everything is great. However, when one doesn't carry out its responsibility, the other needs to get a move on.

You could probably stay to strengthen your center, as well. "The hip flexors connect to the front of the spine and cross over the front of the hip, so if your center is inactive, at that point you will either slump or hyperstretch into your lower back, putting increased pressure on the hip flexors and less action in the glutes," says Heffron. Same issue; diverse trigger.

Spin class and cycling are high on the rundown of guilty parties for making your hip flexors sore, however, it's actually all attached to sitting. Regardless of whether on a seat, on a plane, or at your work area, remaining in a seat most hours of the day puts your hip flexors in a contracted and shortened position while additionally blocking your glutes from working. You are attempting to use your hip flexors when they're tight and this compounds the issue (and, in this manner, raises the pain).

"In no way, shape or form does this mean you have to stay away from a spin class or riding your bicycle," guarantees Heffron. It just means you have to do some additional quality work to battle those muscle imbalances.

Pain in the hip flexor or front of the hip/leg can be related to a few potential causes. At the point when you experience pain in the front of the hip, and it doesn't have an undeniable component of damage, (for example, tripping in a hole while running), at that point, it's quite often dreary movement damage or identified with poor posture and additionally biomechanics.

The area of pain in the hip flexor area can run from mid-thigh to the groin area to the lower stomach (from the gut catch to the PSIS, which is the back predominant iliac spine) or the front of the pelvic bone merely up and horizontal to the groin area where the essential hip flexor (psoas) starts.

Hip Flexor Pain and Pain in the Front of the Hip
Normal potential reasons behind pain in the front of the hip include:

1. Femoral Stress Fracture

2. Hernia

3. Femoral Acetabular Impingement (FAI)

4. Groin Muscle Strain

5. Low Back Pain (LBP)

6. Hip Flexor Strain

I will cover every one of these in more detail.

There are several basic reasons to have pain in or around the hip flexors. Frequently, the reason for the pain is almost identical (overuse). It's critical to get the right conclusion to ensure that you're treating the right areas.

Muscle Strain

Hip flexor strains most generally happen because of an abrupt constriction of the hip flexor muscles (especially in a place of stretch). They regularly happen during sprinting or kicking exercises. This is especially true during dangerous exercises, increasing speed or when a footballer does a long kick, especially following a missing warm-up.

Patients typically feel an abrupt sharp pain or pulling sensation in the front of the hip or groin at the time of damage. In minor strains, the pain might be insignificant, permitting you to proceed with movement. In increasingly extreme cases, patients may experience serious damage, muscle freezing, weakness and a failure to proceed with the action. Patients with an extreme hip flexor strain may likewise be unable to walk without limping.

Patients with this condition usually experience pain while lifting the knee towards the chest (particularly against opposition) or during exercises, for example, running, kicking or going upstairs. It is additionally normal for patients to experience pain or stiffness after these exercises with rest. A hip flexor strain is an injury described as tearing off of at least one of the hip flexor muscles and commonly causes pain in the front of the hip or groin.

The group of muscles at the front of the hip is known as the hip flexors. The most commonly included muscle in a hip flexor strain is the iliopsoas. The hip flexors are responsible for moving the knee towards the chest (for example, twisting the hip) during movement and are especially active when running or kicking. At whatever point the hip flexors contract or are put under strain, the pressure is put through the hip flexor muscle strands.

At the point when this pressure is unnecessary because of an excess of reiteration or high power, the hip flexor muscle strands may tear. At the point when this happens, the condition is known as a hip flexor strain. Tears to the hip flexors can run from a small incomplete tear where there is insignificant pain and a negligible loss of capacity, to a total break including an abrupt incident of extreme pain and significant disability.

Biomechanics

Poor development control can, likewise cause hip flexor pain. This is regularly seen with hip flexor squats. At the point when squats are done inaccurately, hip flexor pain can happen because of weakness in the back gluteal muscles and tightness in the foremost hip flexor muscles. The inability to remain upright during a deep squat shows both an absence of gluteal (butt cheek) quality and tightness in the foremost hip flexors.

A test for tight hip flexors is to lie on your back on the table and let your legs drop over the edge. At that point hold one knee and let the other leg drop down, and if your knee isn't lower than the table, at that point your hip flexor is tight. This is known as the Thomas test.

Both a hip flexor strain and hip pain from poor development examples can be dealt with adequately with physiotherapy.

Femoral Stress Fractures

The femur is the biggest and longest bone in the body. Nonetheless, that doesn't imply it can't cause a stress fracture. Stress fractures are an interesting kind of bone fracture as they sometimes happen because of a particular trauma. Stress fractures regularly happen because of a series of occasions that cause the bone not to have the option to deal with the pressure of your movement, (for example, running) which brings about a split in the bone.

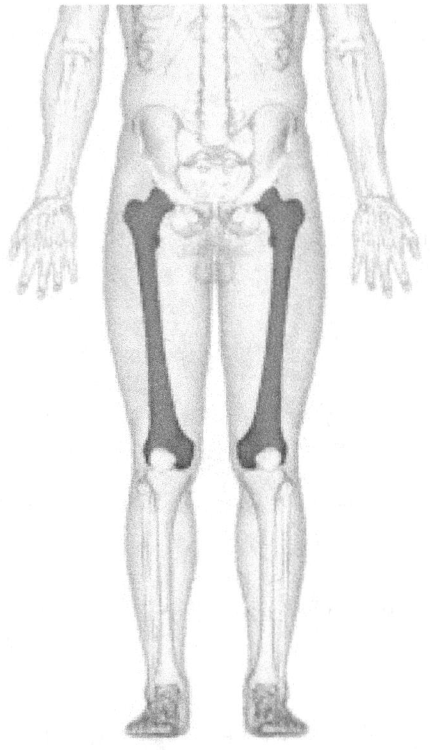

At first, you may scarcely even notice the pain related with a stress fracture; however the pain will in general decline with time. The delicacy ordinarily starts from a particular spot and reduces during rest. As the damage decreases, the pain will in general spread out and turn out to be gradually diffused with a central area of sensitivity. You may have to stretch around the painful area. In cases of femoral stress fractures, the pain will frequently be diffuse and spread throughout the femur or thigh.

At the point when the pile up of more movement are too much for the bone to bear, a stress fracture will happen. By and large, a decrease or complete end to training will at first be essential. It will be important to take close take a look at the occasions that caused the break, including an exhaustive assessment of your running plans and nourishment levels.

Hernia Pain
Pain brought about by a hernia (especially, in the inguinal area) can mimic hip flexor or groin pain.

Indications of Hernia Pain include:

- A little lump on either side of the pelvic bone. The size can change contingent upon movement and particularly, with coughing and straining.
- There might be an exhausting or achy sensation in the crotch region or close to the bugling.

There is expanded pain after movement, including running and weightlifting. Coughing can make it worse.

- There could be a sense of weight or weakness in the groin area.

If you think that you may have a hernia, at that point, it's critical to have it assessed by a medical expert.

Femoral Acetabular Impingement (FAI)

Femoral Acetabular impingement (FAI), otherwise called hip impingement, is the major reason for hip osteoarthritis in individuals younger than 50. FAI is due to bone spurs (bone overgrowth) along with the bones that make up the hip joint. The extra bone causes the bones to have an unpredictable shape and never again fit completely into the ball and attachment joint. The bones begin to rub and squeeze the tissue inside the hip. This will frequently influence the labrum, which is a part of the connection.

- Indications of Femoral Acetabular Impingement (FAI) include:
- Pain (ordinarily in the groin area or potentially toward the outside of the hip).
- Sharp pain with turning, twisting, as well as hunching down in a weight-bearing position.
- Stiffness and a feeling of a dull throb inside the hip joint when very still.
- When FAI indications are relaxed, running may normally give the impression of solidness and achiness with a periodic stabbing pain. As the bones and ligament wear, the symptoms will worsen.

The pain will, in general, shift contingent upon movement levels. It can come and go with extensive periods lacking a lot of issues. The more active you are, the more probable you will produce declining symptoms.

Common Treatment for Femoral Acetabular Impingement (FAI):

- Exercise Modification.
- Anti-Inflammatory Medications.
- Physical Therapy. It tends to be useful to usually try improving your range of movement (ROM) and to strengthen the muscles of your hips and pelvis that help the hip joint. This can, generally, lessen a portion of the weight on the damaged labrum and ligament.

Groin Muscle Strain

A groin strain is generally basic in people associated with running events that require trip cutting and shifting, of course. The quick movement and huge amount of power can cause a strain or draw in the internal thigh and groin musculature. This can also happen to sprinters while trail running. You may need to rapidly alter course on the path or jump over and around an obstacle in the way.

Symptoms of a Groin Muscle Strain include:

- Pain and tenderness in the internal thigh and groin area.
- There is normally a popping sensation during the damage with moderate to serious pain.
- Pain that will, in general, feel somewhat better when somewhat active in straight arranged importance advances or in reverse (sagittal) movement, however it can turn out to be extremely sharp and damaging with any speedy developments or as the force increases.
- The pain will, in general, be deep and throbbing in the groin area after the action.

- Pain when you join your legs together (hip adduction) or oppose this movement.

- Pain when you raise your knee and flex your hip.

The underlying treatment for a crotch strain/pull is PRICE (Protection, Rest, Ice, Compression, and Elevation).

Potential Treatments for a Groin Muscle Strain:

- Anti-inflammatories.

- Acupuncture.

- **Soft Tissue Mobilization**. Slow, direct, and gentle weight over the painful areas can be useful to elevate pain and tightness. Back massage treatment or using a froth roller (or other preparation instrument) around the encompassing areas may also be useful.

- **Exercise**. When you begin to stretch and exercise the area, it is essential to focus on recapturing full hip and pelvic mobility without pain and for the most part chipping away at center adjustment just as internal thigh and hip reinforcing exercises. Progressing all the more gradually is quite often prompted with these injuries.

Low Back Pain (LBP)

One may look at the first miracle of why low back pain (LBP) is recorded as a potential reason behind pain in the front of the hip or hip flexor. However, pain in the hip flexors and front of the hip can frequently be related to LBP.

The biggest muscle group that flexes the hip is the psoas major and minor. These two muscles begin on the front part of the spine somewhere inside the stomach area from the twelfth thoracic vertebrae and lumbar vertebrae L5-L1. This implies any issue affecting the spine can also cause pain for these two hip flexor muscles. Moreover, pain in the spine will, in general, refer to pain to different areas of the pelvis and lower leg dependent upon where the pain begins. The pain might be legitimately over the damaged area.

Hip Flexor Strain

There are numerous regular reasons for pain in the front of the thigh. Pain in the hip flexors themselves can also be a confusing route. There are a few muscles that flex the hip, including the psoas major and minor; iliacus; sartorius; and the rectus femoris (one of the quadriceps muscles). Regularly with a genuine hip flexor strain, it's normal to have various muscle groups damaged or affected.

The two most basic reasons to have hip flexor pain is a traumatic strain or abuse damage (normally because of broken biomechanics or potentially postural brokenness).

Symptoms of a Hip Flexor Strain include:

- A sudden and sharp pain/pulling in the front of the hip at the time of damage. Contingent upon the seriousness, you might have the option to finish your movement.
- As the pain worsens, there is generally an impression of deep achiness. Related muscle spasms and weakness are available.
- In increasingly serious cases, an individual will limp and have a notably shorter walk length.

- Pain while lifting the knee/flexing the hip is more terrible with opposition.
- Stretching will at first help decrease the pain, yet it will rapidly return as an individual proceeds with upstanding movement.
- Notable pain and stiffness (especially before anything else or after prolonged sitting and rest).

On account of abuse damage, pain in the hip flexors will intensify as movement level and force increases and will increase normally after some time. Pain first experienced toward the start of a run can halfway settle halfway during the run. At that point, the pain will gradually increase and raise as the run advances. It gets worse the longer and accelerates as you go. Stretching the hip flexor will have a soothing constructive outcome, yet it's normally fleeting. This is progressively basic with perpetual issues, for example, tendinitis.

Handle the issue with information so you can decide whether your customers truly have tight hips or if there is another issue. With a couple of new stretches and exercises, you can help those with tight hip flexors relax them, show signs of improving mobility with less pain, and keep away from injuries.

What Exactly Are Tight Hip Flexors?

To start with, help your customers understand what the hip flexors are, their main cause, and how you recognize when they're tight. The term hip flexors alludes to a group of muscles in and around the hips that help move the legs and the trunk together, like when you lift your leg up, bowing at the hip.

The Hip Flexor Muscle Group

The hip flexor incorporates:

- The iliopsoas, which is two muscles, the psoas and the iliacus,
- The tensor fasciae latae,
- The rectus femoris,
- And the sartorius.

Together these muscles produce flexion, the expansion and overhauling of muscles that take into consideration flexing of the hip joint. They also help to balance out the spine.

Strengthening the center is imperative to supporting the hip flexors, yet are sit-ups the ideal approach to work your abs? We have the appropriate response here.

Signs You Have Tight Hip Flexors
The obvious sign is that these muscles feel tight. You try to stretch them, and they don't move a lot. In any case, there are different signs as well. Tight hip flexor muscles can affect a few different areas of your body so that you may have:

- Tightness or pain in your lower back, particularly when standing.
- Poor posture and trouble standing upright.
- Neck tightness and pain.
- Pain in the glutes.

You can also do a test to assess tightness. Lying on your back on a table or seat, pull one knee up toward your chest and hold it there. Let the other leg loosen up descending over the edge of the table. It helps here to have somebody hold that leg for you so you can do it gradually. If your hip flexors are fine, you should be able to completely expand the thigh so its parallel to the floor and twist the knee to 90 degrees without the thigh rising. Any trouble with these events shows tight hip flexor muscles.

What Causes Hip Tightness?

For most people, the biggest reason for tightness is our main issue throughout the day: sitting for a long time is a significant cause of tightening up the hip flexors. At the point when you sit throughout the day at a work area, the iliopsoas, specifically, shortens, making the flexors tight.

Some athletes are additionally increasingly inclined to tightness. Sprinters use the hip flexors, particularly the iliopsoas, to lift the leg up with each walk. This continued shortening of the muscle isn't compensated by a lengthening expansion. Sprinters frequently end up with tight hip flexors consequently.

Having a weak core can also be an issue that adds to tight hip flexors. Since these muscles are associated with and settle the spine, they frequently assume control over when the center isn't stable. This can prompt pain and tightening.

Why Weak Hip Flexors Can Be a Pain

Pigeon and other hip-opening stances may feel extraordinary while you're in them, however regularly the help is just temporary. If so for you, do you ever address why these deep muscles feel so tight constantly? They could be making up for weak or inhibited hip flexors.

Regardless of whether you think about yourself as a functioning individual and do yoga, odds are you additionally invest a great deal of energy sitting. Excess sitting can make hip flexors shorten and decrease the capacity of muscles and belt to skim against one another during expansion. To more readily see how these significant hip flexors can impact your rear, we should investigate the life systems.

The powerful ILIOPSOAS muscle is frequently referred to as one, yet is really two distinct muscles; the iliacus and the psoas. The iliopsoas ventures north from the lesser trochanter on the upper inward thigh bone and cross the edge of the pelvis. However, from that point the iliacus inserts into the iliac peak and the psoas on the spine, which gives them marginally various capacities. Tenacity between these two muscles can bring about one of them (regularly the iliacus) tiring and both (particularly the psoas) becoming less effective.

The PSOAS is a powerful flexor of the hip joint, however perhaps significantly more critically, it's a unique stabilizer of the lumbar spine. Associating your legs to the lower back, the psoas inserts into the bodies and transverse procedures of the considerable number of vertebrae of the lumbar spine to help the bend of the lower back on the two sides.

ILIACUS covers the entire average surface of your hip bones and connects with the sacroiliac joint. This profound layer of muscle needs to connect right off the bat in growth to balance out both the hip joint and the SI-joint.

As should be obvious, the hip flexors move the legs, yet in addition they balance out the pelvis and lower back. They should be both supple and strong.

Supporting the hip joint from behind are the EXTERNAL ROTATORS, regularly referred to as 'the profound six' which are situated in your seat. These are the muscles you focus on pigeon present. You have hidden the ground-breaking GLUTEUS MAXIMUS, your most important hip extensor that forms the shape of your hip, these moderately small, yet significant six muscles only back to the hip joint interface the sacrum and the lower end of the spine to the highest point of the thigh bones. These deep six are the piriformis, the obturator internus and externus, the gemellus prevalent and substandard, and the quadratus femoris. The PIRIFORMIS, the biggest of the six, also interfaces with the SI-joint and balances out the pelvis on the legs in weight bearing-presents.

There is a significant association between the psoas and the piriformis since they bolster the lower some portion of the spine both vertically and on a level plane. If the psoas is underactive and the iliacus overworked, the smaller stabilizers in the back will attempt to make up for the subsequent absence of soundness in the area.

Making an interpretation of The Anatomy to Your Practice
In our yoga practice, it can be enticing to concentrate on hip adaptability, and disregard the similarly significant strengthening and balancing out work. So regardless of whether your hip flexors feel tight, that doesn't mean they have to get longer. Most yogis have all that could be needed range of movement in hip augmentation. Much of the time, the hip flexor muscles need assembling and strengthening more than they need stretching.

And, similarly as stretching the hip flexors can be counterproductive, so can discharging those tight outer rotators without taking care of the hidden issue of restraint or weakness. Ensuring your iliopsoas is solid and useful could after some time decrease the heap on those grumpy rotators in the back and even improve your scope of movement.

Key Points

- There is a contrast between a quadriceps stretch and a hip flexor stretch. At the point when your method of reasoning for doing the stretch is to try stretching your hip flexor, focus on the psoas and not the rectus femoris.

- Keep it to a one joint stretch. Many individuals need to hop right to play out a hip flexor stretch while flexing the knee. This joins the rectus and the psoas, yet I find far too many individuals cannot fittingly do this stretch. They will redress, for the most part by stretching their front vessel to an extreme or hyper stretching their lumbar spine.

- Stay tall. Fight the temptation to incline toward the stretch and truly expand your hip. A great many people are unreasonably tight due to this; trust me. You'll wind up loosening up the foremost hip joint and abs more than the hip flexor.

- Make sure you fuse a back, pelvic tilt. Arrange your abs and your glutes to work out a back, pelvic tilt. This will give you the "genuine" stretch we are searching for while choosing this stretch. Many individuals won't even need to lean in a bit; they'll feel it promptly in the front of their hip.

- If you don't feel it, squeeze your glutes harder. Many individuals make some hard memories spinning on their glutes while doing this stretch, yet it is critical.

- If despite everything you don't feel it, lean in only a bit. If you are certain your glutes and abs are squeezed, and you are in back, pelvic tilt and still don't feel it much, lean in only a couple of inches. Our first movement of this is easy to lean forward in 1-3 inches; however, keep your pelvis in back tilt.

- Guide your hips with your hands. I generally start this stretch with your hands on your hips so I can instruct you to feel back a pelvic tilt. Spot your fingers in the front and thumbs in the back and sign them to back tilt and make their thumbs descend.

- Progress to include core engagement. When they can ace the back, pelvic tilt, I, for the most part, progress to helping by restoring core engagement, you can do this by pacing two hands together over your front knee and drive straight down, or by holding a back massage stick or dowel before you and pushing down into the ground. Key here is to have the arms straight and to push down with your core, not your triceps.

Issues with Hip Core Retraining

Other than not having a popular name yet, the hip center can be effectively retrained; however, it is increasingly hard to identify which muscles they are. Also, you will have the variable hip core capacity to your left side compared with your right.

Much the same as with lower back core exercises it is important not to advance too rapidly. If you over-burden the muscle, it will essentially quit working or lose control, leading to expanded possibility of injury.

What to Do?

If you have endured hip or crotch pain that keeps on nagging you, it likely could be because of a "poor hip core." Your PCP may have diagnosed you as having trochanteric bursitis, which is possible injury brought about by hip instability. While an infusion may help facilitate the short-term symptoms, they will in general return because your "hip core" reacts to restorative exercises, not infusion!

If so, at that point, please get in touch with us to have your hip core evaluated. Your Physio can do a full hip and pelvis appraisal and start you on medicinal treatment straight away.

PhysioWorks has structured a remedial "hip center adjustment" program to assist you with defeating hip and groin pain quickly. Besides, for the individuals who experience issues feeling your right muscles working, we can use an ultrasound scanner to outwardly assist you with finding your hip core and see them in real life.

Normal Hip Pain Treatment Options

- Early Injury Treatment
- Avoid the HARM Factors

What to do after a Muscle Strain or Ligament Sprain?

- Acupuncture and Dry Needling
- Sub-Acute Soft Tissue Injury Treatment
- Core Exercises
- Closed Kinetic Chain Exercises
- Active Foot Posture correction Exercises

- Gait Analysis

- Biomechanical Analysis

- Balance Enhancement Exercises

- Proprioception and Balance Exercises

- Agility and Sport-Specific Exercises

- Medications

- Orthotics

- Real-Time Ultrasound Physiotherapy

- Soft Tissue Massage

- Brace or Support

- Dry Needling

- Electrotherapy and Local Modalities

- Heat Packs

- Joint Mobilization Techniques

- Kinesiology Tape

- Neurodynamics

- Prehabilitation

- Running Analysis

- Strength Exercises

- Stretching Exercises

- Supportive Taping & Strapping

- TENS Machine

- Video Analysis

- Yoga

Hip Related Conditions

General Information

- Hip Pain

- Groin Pain

Hip Joint Pain

- Hip Arthritis - Osteoarthritis

- Hip Labral Tear

- Hip Pointer

- Femoroacetabular Impingement - FAI

- Perthes Disease

- Slipped Femoral Capital Epiphysis

- Stress Fracture

- Avascular Necrosis of the Femoral Head

Parallel Hip Pain

- Gluteal Tendinopathy

- Greater Trochanteric Pain Syndrome

- Trochanteric Bursitis

Adductor-related Groin Pain

- Adductor Tendinopathy

- Groin Strain

Pubic-related Groin Pain

- Osteitis Pubis

Inguinal-related Groin Pain

- Inguinal hernia

- Sportsman's hernia

Iliopsoas-related Groin Pain

- Hip Flexor Strain

Other Muscle-related Pain

- Piriformis Syndrome

- Muscle Pain - Muscle Strain

- Poor Hip Core

- DOMS - Delayed Onset Muscle Soreness

- Cramps

- Core Stability Deficiency

Systemic Diseases

- Rheumatoid Arthritis

- Fibromyalgia

- Osteoporosis

Referred Sources

- Sacroiliac Joint Pain - SIJ

- Sciatica

- Lower Back Pain

- Pinched Nerve

Hip Surgery

- Hip Replacement

Reasons for hip issues

There are many conditions that may mess hip up, for example,

- Osteoarthritis

- Rheumatoid joint pain

- Ankylosing spondylitis

- Bone breaks

- Developmental dysplasia of the hip

- Perthes' infection

- Slipped capital femoral epiphysis

- Irritable hip disorder.

Osteoarthritis

Osteoarthritis is related to degeneration of the joint cartilage and with changes during the bones fundamental the joint. The ligament gets fragile and parts. A few parts may split away and skim around inside the synovial liquid inside the joint. This can lead to inflammation.

In the end, the cartilage can separate then it never pads the two bones again. Current theory suggests the cartilage loses its mobility on account of cell changes. Generally affected joints include those of the hip, spine, shoulder, fingers, knees, lower legs, feet and toes.

Rheumatoid arthritis

Rheumatoid arthritis is an insusceptible condition that causes inflammation in moving joints (synovial joints).

In spite of the fact that individuals who end up with rheumatoid joint inflammation may have an inclination to the condition, the 'trigger' for creating indications is unknown.

Inflammation in joints brings about an expansion in synovial liquid (expanding of the joint), pain and morning joint stiffness. Joints that can be affected incorporate those of the hands and wrists, elbows, shoulders, neck, jaw, hips, knees, lower legs and feet.

Ankylosing spondylitis

This exceptional type of incendiary joint inflammation can focus on the spine, knees and hips. Regular symptoms include pain and stiffness first thing for the morning. The reason is unknown. However, qualities should assume a critical job.

Ankylosing spondylitis can happen without anyone else or in relationship with a different issue, including Crohn's disease, ulcerative colitis and psoriasis. Caucasian men aged somewhere in the range of 16 and 33 years are generally susceptible.

Bone fracture

More seasoned individuals are increasingly inclined to hip breaks since bones become less thick as we age. Sometimes, an individual develops osteoporosis, an infection described by excessive loss of bone tissue. The bones become delicate and fragile and inclined to breaks and deformations. A larger number of ladies than men experience osteoporosis.

Developmental dysplasia of the hip

Developmental dysplasia of the hip means that the hip joint of a newborn baby is disengaged or inclined to separation. The connection is unusually shallow, which prevents a steady fit. Slack ligaments may also enable the femoral head to slip out of joint.

Potential causes incorporate a breech (feet first) delivery, family ancestry and disorders, for example, spine bifida. Around 95 percent of children born with formative dysplasia of the hip can be effectively treated.

Perthes' disease

Perthes' disease is an illness of the hip joint. It will, in general, affect kids between the ages of three and 11 years. The head of the femur is softened, and eventually damaged, because of a deficient blood supply deep down in the cells.

Most youngsters with Perthes' illness, in the end, recuperate. However, it can take somewhere in the range of two to five years for the femoral head to recover. The reason is unknown.

Slipped capital femoral epiphysis

During childhood, the femoral ball is attached to the femur with a growth plate of bone. In certain adolescents, the ball can slide from its legitimate position, making the leg on the affected side deflect out from the body.

Possible contributing elements incorporate the shape and area of the femoral head in connection to the femur, increased sex hormones during pubescence, and weight gain. Without treatment, slipped capital femoral epiphysis will worsen, and the kid may experience joint pain of the hip joint in later life.

Irritable hip syndrome

Irritable hip syndrome (sometimes called harmful synovitis) is a temporary type of joint pain, which will in general influence prepubescent children for obscure reasons. Young men with lethal synovitis dwarf young ladies four to one. Side effects incorporate hip pain (normally on one side in particular), failure to walk (or limping), knee pain and fever. Most instances of poisonous synovitis resolve without help inside half a month.

Soft tissue pain and referred pain

Pain that can have all the earmarks of being originated from the hip joint and may be identified with soft tissue structures around the hip, for example, muscles, tendons and bursae, or might be referred from a back issue. Pain experienced over the side of the hip might be expected to be trochanteric bursitis.

Diagnosing hip issues

Contingent upon the reason, finding of a hip issue can include various tests including:

- Medical history
- Physical assessment
- X-beams

- Ultrasound checks

- Bone checks

- Biopsy

- Blood tests.

Treatment choices for hip issues

There are different treatment choices for hip issues, contingent upon the basic reason:

- For all types of joint pain, there are non-pharmacological treatment choices, medicines that don't include prescriptions, for example, exercise programs, instruction and self-administration programs. Explicit medications are accessible for various sorts of joint inflammation. For osteoarthritis, the most well-known kind of joint inflammation, basic pain-relieving medicine is regularly viable. Joint replacement medical procedure (hip or knee) might be the best choice for individuals with serious osteoarthritis

- Rheumatoid joint pain and ankylosing spondylitis, for the most part, require increasingly complex treatment, for example, anti-inflammatory medications and disease-modifying medicines. A few people may likewise require surgeries.

- Fracture treatment incorporates admission to a clinic and medical procedures.

- For babies with formative dysplasia of the hip an extraordinary outfit is worn for somewhere in the range of six and 12 weeks to hold the joint in place while the infant's skeleton grows and develops

- Perthes' disease – Choices include bed rest, pain-reducing drugs, support or brace (worn for somewhere in the range of one and two years to resources for re-attaching the femoral head to sit inside the connection) and medical procedure to treat deformities.

- Slipped capital femoral epiphysis – The medical procedure can reposition the femoral head and screw it strongly into the right spot.

- Irritable hip disorder – Choices incorporate bed rest, pain easing drugs and non-steroidal anti-inflammatory medications (NSAIDs)

- Soft tissue pain – Neighborhood symptomatic estimates, for example, an exercise program, calming creams and basic pain decreasing prescriptions may enable delicate tissue to pain.

Exercises

Double Banded Pull Through

- Attach a long opposition band low to the ground behind you. Or then again, you can also use a cable.

- Stand before the band with your feet about shoulder-width separated with a circle smaller than expected opposition band simply over your knees. Push your legs separated somewhat to effectively keep up strain in the band and keep your knees from caving in.

- Lean forward at the hips and drive your butt back as you twist your knees to reach down and snatch the long band between your legs. You should feel a stretch in your hamstrings and glutes.

- Keep your chest lifted and back level as you remain back up, driving your hips forward and pressing your glutes at the top. That is 1 rep.

- Do 12-15 reps.

Side Plank with Knee Drive

"The energetic exercise of the moving leg adds a considerably more prominent test to the base glutes attempting to isometrically hold the bodyweight in that strong position," says Miranda.

- Start at the side board with your left elbow under your shoulder, legs expanded, and hips, knees, and lower legs stacked. Draw in your center, fold your butt, and ensure your lower back is level.
- Slowly drive your right knee up toward your chest. Delay for a second, and then gradually stretch out the leg and pull it out to the beginning position. That is 1 rep.
- Do 5-8 reps on every leg.

Banded Hip March

- Stand upright with your feet about hip-width separated, center drawn in, and chest lifted, with a circle smaller than a normal obstruction band around the balls of the two feet.
- Slowly drive your right knee up and out before you, halting when it arrives at hip height. (You will be unable to lift that high by relying upon your present mobility.) You should feel your hip flexors in the lifted leg working, and your glutes on the balancing out leg working.
- Focus on keeping your foot legitimately under your knee, your pelvis level, and your standing-leg knee, hip, and lower leg in line.
- Slowly let your leg down. That is 1 rep.
- Do 5-8 reps on every leg, exchanging sides.

Bulgarian Split Squat

- Stand with your back to a seat or comparative raised surface. With your left foot on the floor a couple of feet before the seat, place the highest point of your right foot on the seat, shoelaces down. Hold a free weight in each hand by your sides.

- Brace your center and twist your knees to drop down into a split squat. Your left knee should perfectly form a 90-degree edge with the goal that your thigh is parallel to the ground, and your right knee is hovering over the floor. (Quick position check: your left foot should be moved out far enough that you can do this without releasing your left knee past your left toes. If you can't, bounce your other foot somewhat more distant away from the seat.)

- Driving through your left heel, get back up to the beginning position. That is 1 rep.

- Do 12-15 reps on each leg.

Step Up to Reverse Lunge

Miranda considers this a "compound mix" move. "It's a term and methodology that I structured that includes stacking together two distinct multi-joint exercises and consolidating them into one movement." It's an amazing method to build the force of exercise without including weight, she includes.

- Stand facing a box, step, seat, or seat.

- Step onto the crate with your right foot and drive through your right impact point and glutes to bring your left leg over to meet the right. Let your left foot drift, and keep the greater part of the weight on your right foot.

- Step back with your left foot, at that point step your right foot back about two feet behind the left and drop down promptly into a reverse lunge.
- Push through your left foot to get back up (that is 1 rep) and move directly into the subsequent stage up.
- Do 12-15 reps on every leg.

6 Hand weight Sumo Squat

- Choose a hand weight that lets you squat with proper form; however, it makes you feel exhausted before the finish of each set.
- Stand with feet more extensive than shoulder-width apart; toes marginally turned out. Hold the dumbbell with two hands at your chest.
- Bend your knees and drop down into a squat.
- Push through your heels to come back to standing and crush your glutes at the top. That is 1 rep.
- Do 8-10 reps.

Kickstand Romanian Deadlift

- Stand with feet hip-width apart, one foot around six steps before the other. Place a free weight (or portable weight) by the two feet.
- The dominant part of your weight should be on your front leg. Rise onto the toes of your back foot, using it as a kickstand to help keep up your balance yet just putting a little weight on it.
- Lean forward at the hips, drive your glutes back, and bring down the weights toward the floor. Keep your back level, and shoulders apart; don't lean forward or curve your lower back.

- Press through your front foot to come back to the beginning position. That is 1 rep.

- Do 5-8 reps on each leg.

Explosive Sprinters Lunge

- Stand tall with your feet hip-width apart.

- Step your right foot back a couple of feet into a tilted position.

- Push through your left foot to dangerously hopping into the air, driving your right knee toward your chest.

- Land with a soft knee (that is 1 rep) and venture back quickly into another lurch.

- Do 5-8 reps on each leg.

Banded Jump Squat

- Place a round smaller than usual opposition band simply over your knees. Remain with your feet about shoulder-width apart.

- Lean forward at your hips and put your butt once more into a squat. Squat as deep as your mobility will permit, however not more distant than parallel to the ground.

- Jump out of sight as high as you can and fix your legs. Swing your arms somewhere near your sides for force, and keep your back straight and chest lifted.

- Land back on the floor with soft knees. That is 1 rep.

- Do 8-10 reps.

Kettlebell Swing

- Stand with your feet shoulder-width apart, a kettlebell on the floor in the middle of your legs.

- Lean forward and twist your knees to crouch and grab the kettlebell handle with two hands.

- Swing the kettlebell between your legs, and afterwards, get back up and use the force from your hips to swing the weight to chest height. Press your butt at the highest point of the movement.

- Immediately drop down as you swing the kettlebell between your legs again to begin the following rep.

- Do 10-12 reps.

Lateral Lunge

- Stand with your feet together, holding a free weight in each hand, arms by your sides.

- Make a major advance (around 2 feet) out to one side. At the point when your foot hits the ground, lean forward at the hips, drive your butt back, and twist your right knee to bring it down into a lurch. The loads should outline your right knee, and your left leg should be straight.

- Pause for a second, and afterwards push off your right leg to come back to the beginning position. Repeat on the other leg. That is 1 rep.

- Do 10-12 reps.

12 Banded Marching Hip Bridge

- Loop a smaller than expected opposition band around the balls of your feet and lie face up before a seat, seat, or step. Place your heels on the seat.
- Push through your heels and press your glutes to lift your hips off the floor. Keep your back level and center locked in.
- Slowly drive your right knee toward your chest, stop for a second, and then place your foot back on the seat. Repeat with your left leg. That is 1 rep.
- Do 10-12 reps.

The Source of All (Efficient) Movement

The hip flexors are a group of muscles around the upper and internal thighs and pelvic area that help control each movement we make. Running, hopping, and even simply standing requires proper flexion and stabilization of the hip flexors.

Strong hip flexors are particularly significant for energetic individuals and athletes, as studies have demonstrated connections between weak hip flexor balancing out muscles and injuries (1).

Why do the hip flexors matter? Not just in light of the fact that a great many people don't concentrate on strengthening their flexors, yet additionally because consistently we do things that both weaken and shorten (or fix) them.

For instance, if you sit before a PC or at a work area for quite a long time every day, it both shortens and fixes the muscles in the front of the body (including your hip flexors). It additionally makes your shoulders round forward, alongside a forward-head posture (2).

And then if go to the rec center for an exercise session after sitting at the work area throughout the day and you don't loosen up and strengthen your hip flexors, you can intensify that terrible stance, causing muscle imbalances.

How does this occur? Since you're preparing muscles while they're in the off base position.

Even Athletes Must Strengthen Hip Flexors

Also, regardless of whether an individual is an athlete (such as a sprinter) who is moving the greater part of the day, they can also be in danger of injuries coming from weak hip flexors.

This is because by not doing exercises that fortify the stabilizer muscles in the hip flexors that keep the pelvis in line, they set themselves up for ill-advised situating of the hips. This would then be able to prompt hip and knee injuries by developing an unstable foot position while running.

That is because the deep muscles of the hip (such as piriformis and quadratus femoris) assume a basic job in hip adjustment (3).

Also, runners with iliotibial band disorder (a typical issue influencing a "band" of muscle that runs from your hip to your knee) had critical weakness in muscles of the hip.

To put it plainly, strengthening the flexors will help keep you away from sway injuries in the lower body by improving the right foot position.

The exact opposite thing you need to do is run a long-distance race (if you do that kind of thing) with inappropriate form. Ouch!

Different Benefits of Strengthening Hip Flexors

Strengthening and increasing hip flexor adaptability can also increase performance. For instance, one study found athletes who did hip flexor exercises as a major part of their routine both improved their hip flexion quality by 12.2 percent and cut their run times by as much as 9 percent.

Also, strengthening those muscles can likewise improve the range of movement, which is additionally pivotal to avoiding injuries.

Since we've found how significant your hip flexors are, how about we take a look at five hip flexor strengthening exercises you can acquaint with your everyday exercise. Realise that a couple of these will require a dependability ball.

5 Exercises to Strengthen Your Hip Flexors

Ball Pikes

While generally, a stomach exercise, ball pikes also require a ton of hip strength to keep up parity and maneuver your hips into a pike position.

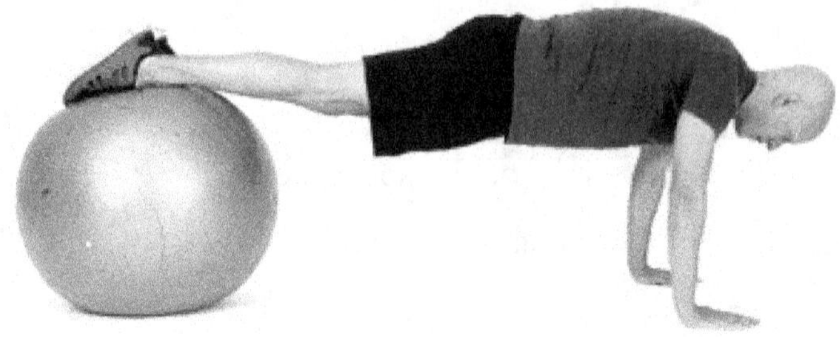

The most effective way to Do Ball Pikes

1.   Begin in a high board position, hands below your shoulders.

2.   Place the highest points of the two feet and shins on your exercise ball.

3.   Raise your hips toward the sky until simply the very tips of your toes are contacting the ball.

4.   Slowly go lower, coming back to the beginning position.

5.   Repeat for 10 to 15 reps, being certain to keep your abs connected through the whole exercise.

Knee Drive Holds

Knee drive holds connect with the hip flexors to drive the knee to the chest, making them a fantastic hip flexor strengthener. You can use either a stability ball or seat for your surface for this exercise.

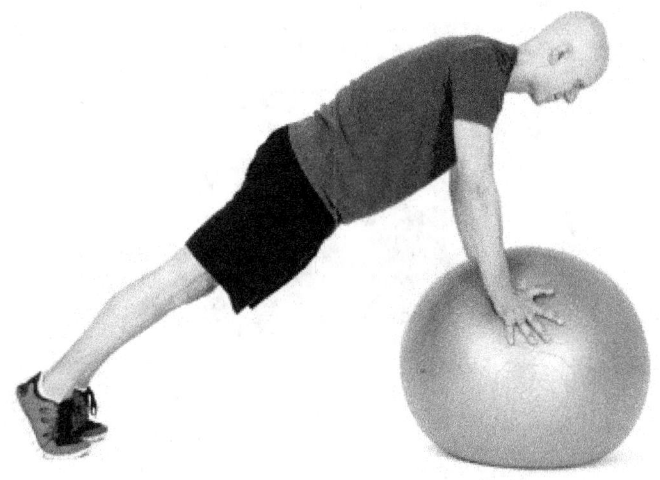

1. The most effective method to Do Knee Drive Holds

2. Begin in a raised push-up position on your seat or ball.

3. Keeping your body in a straight line from head to toe, with your abs connected, drive one knee in toward your chest.

4. Hold your knee set up for a 2-to 3-second check.

5. Return to your push-up position and continue using the other leg.

6. Repeat for 10 to 12 reps.

Dead Bug

The dead bug is another exercise that connects with the hip flexors, this time in both an isometric hold as you broaden your leg, and withdrawal as you return your leg to a parallel position.

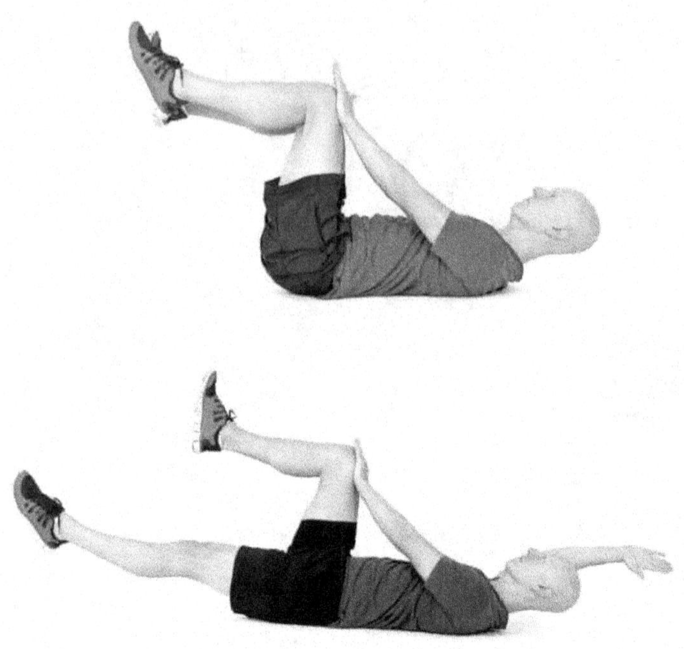

The most effective way to do the Dead Bug

1. Begin lying on the floor on your back. Connecting with your abs, raise your legs off the floor at a 90-degree point.

2. Now, expand and bring down your right leg until it's only a couple of steps off the floor, while at the same time raising your left arm over your head.

3. Hold for a 2-second tally.

4. Now, take your stretched leg and arm back to the beginning position and repeat on the opposite side.

5. Aim for 10 to 15 reps.

Reverse Lunge with Knee Drive

The reverse lunge with knee drive gives a powerful stretch to the hip flexors while likewise fortifying them as you drive your knee toward your chest.

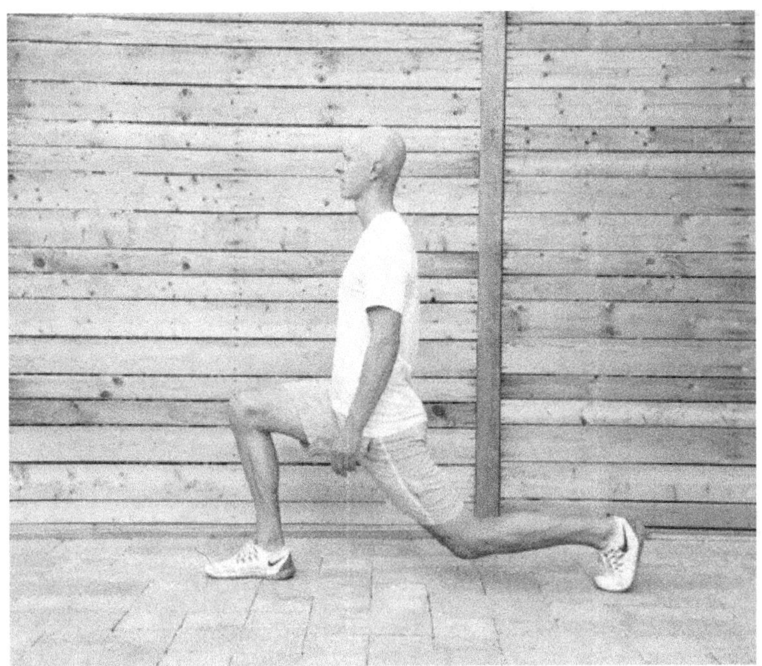

Step by step instructions to do the Reverse Lunge with Knee Drive

1. Begin standing tall, feet hip-width apart.

2. Stretch your right leg back behind you and lower your body into a lunge on your front leg.

3. Now draw in your glutes and push back to standing, however, rather than restoring your foot to the floor, drive your knee in toward your chest.

4. This knee drive should take a two-second pause to rely on the raise and lower; don't attempt to drive the knee too rapidly.

5. Return to your beginning position and repeat on the other leg.

6. Aim for 10 to 15 reps.

Ball Knee Tucks

Ball knee tucks are like ball pikes. However, rather than lifting our hips toward the sky, we're keeping them level and using the lower abs and hip flexors to pull our knees in toward our chest.

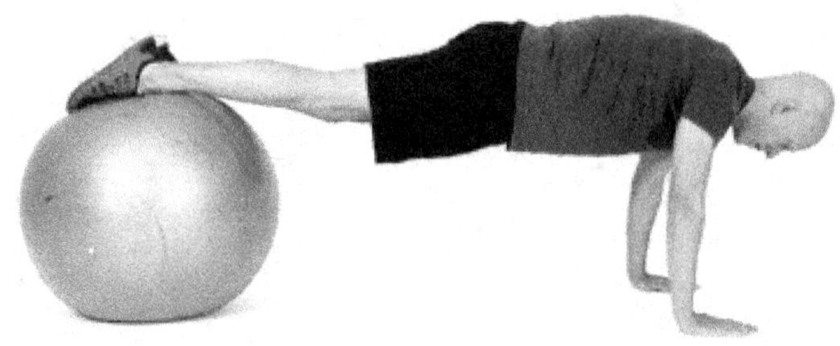

Instructions to Do Ball Knee Tucks

1. Begin in a push-up position, the highest points of your feet and shins on your ball.

2. Keeping your middle parallel to the ground, draw both your knees in toward your chest.

3. Slowly come back to your beginning position and repeat, avoiding shaking your body to and fro as you complete the movement.

4. Aim for 10 to 15 reps.

Stretching is Important Too

While these exercises are extraordinary for strengthening the hip flexors, it's additionally significant that we take a shot at their adaptability.

That is because tight hip flexors can add to bad posture, which causes an entire host of medical issues all by itself, however, "pulling down" the chest area. This is particularly valid for the individuals who go through a large portion of their days sitting down or work at a PC.

To battle tight hip flexors, try this simple stretch you can do anyplace:

1. Begin by staying in a lunge position, right foot forward.
2. Lower your left knee to the ground and drive your hips forward marginally until you feel a stretch somewhere down in your hamstrings.
3. Hold for 20 to 30 seconds, at that point switch legs.

Try Foam Rolling

It might also be helpful to foam roll your hip flexors a few times each week, particularly if they feel tight after delayed sitting.

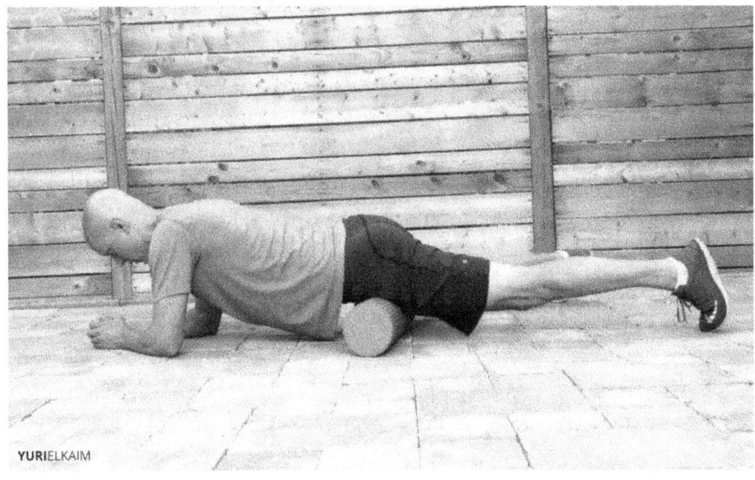

Here's an extraordinary move for the hip flexors:

1. Facing down, drop your hips onto the froth roller, completely stretching the legs.
2. Lean-to the side you need to take a shot at, using the toes on your opposite leg for balance.
3. Repeat on the opposite side.

Solid Hips, Happy Body

With these exercises to strengthen hip flexors, you'll be standing and running tall and strong in the blink of an eye.

But remember, consistency is the key — it requires some investment to beat incessant snugness from long stretches of sitting.

You may have been informed that the appropriate response is to experience a flood of clumsy hip flexor stretches as frequently as could be allowed. In truth, that is just a part of the deal. Similarly, as with the shoulder, you have to crush, stretch, and fortify your hip flexors to improve them.

Come Unglued

The initial phase in building better hip flexors is to go through some difficult minutes disturbing tissues that have been frozen from long periods of sitting at a work area. I prescribe rolling, otherwise known as "self-myofascial discharge."

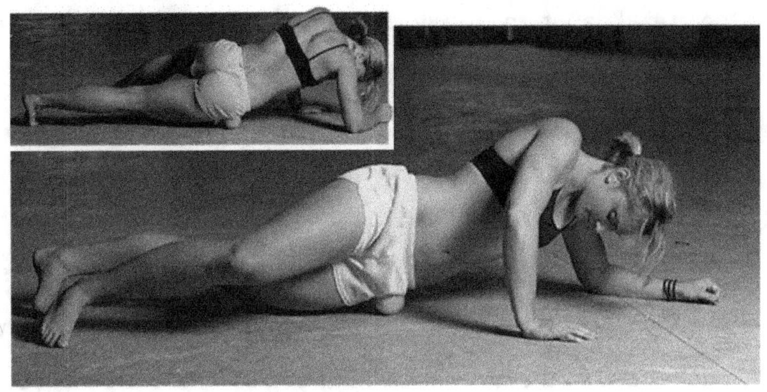

You can move on pretty much anything. I've used a few unique kinds of froth rollers, a Rumble Roller, lacrosse balls, PVC pipe, and various odd stick-shaped things. I've also been getting extraordinary outcomes using the Body Wrench, an amazing gadget that is essentially a mix of the entirety of the above mentioned. I have found that various materials are reasonable for various zones on various bodies, so don't hesitate to try and find what works best for you. Continue changing your position until you locate a problem area, and then hold that position for in any event 30 seconds.

To work these tissues, start by finding your iliac crest. Sounds like rare bird's species. However, it's the top hard part of your hip that sticks out by your beltline. In case you're using a lacrosse ball, essentially move into a board position on the ground and lay on the ball with the goal that it presses into your hip just beneath the peak. Move side-to-side gradually, so the ball moves back and forth, laterally several inches at a time.

Continue altering your position until you locate a problem area ("A what? I don't have a clue what you're ... Gracious! My God! There one is!"), and then hold that position for at least 30 seconds. Your first drive will be to worry when you feel tenderness, yet it's significant that you unwind and keep on moving around the area. Keep it up, and don't rush. The more gradually and all the more frequently you can do this, the better.

Jump on the Couch

Since we smoothed out that old tissue and dislodged a couple of fossilized nasties, we should perceive what we can do about improving extensibility. The couch stretch is one of the best movements you can do for opening up your hip to the end range of movement. Take a kneeling position before something that you can use to hold your foot up (i.e., a love seat). Your back knee should be flexed, which means your heel is as close as conceivable to your butt.

It's anything but difficult to repay in this position by hyper stretching your lower back, however, it's pivotal that you don't. Rather, I need you to concentrate on pressing your glutes and hamstrings, which will drive your hips forward into an all-out "schwing." If your right foot is back, you should feel an exceptional stretch on the right front side of your hip. Hold it for quite a while, similar to a moment or two, and then switch sides.

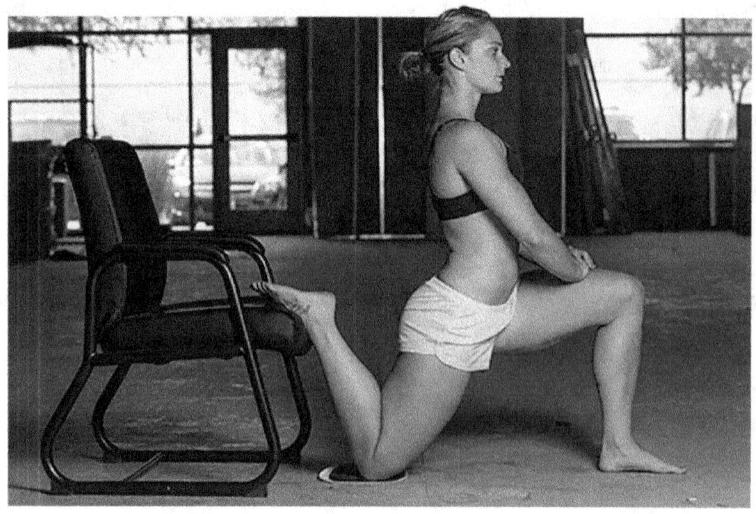

Like moving, this is a development that should be done as regularly as you can tolerate. Physical specialist and mentor Kelly Starrett has written that you should do it for two minutes on each side each half-hour. That might be difficult to manage. However, the fact of the matter is this: Frequent, long-span stretches are the main stretches that will have any noteworthy impact on your tissue length and portability. If you want to get better, you need to surrender.

Build Flexible Flexors

At the point when I initially started preparing, I accepted that since I had short, tight hip flexors, they should be strong. Wrong! Since we spend such a large amount of our lives sitting, a position wherein the hip flexors are latently contracted, many people's flexors are both short and weak.

The psoas, our essential hip flexor, is typically the weakest of the five flexors, and the other four hip flexors need to work more subsequently. To test if it's so for you, lift one knee well over 90 degrees and hold it there, guaranteeing that you don't cheat by pushing your pelvis or inclining ahead. If holding this for more than a couple of moments is painful or impossible for you, your psoas suck. You will experience genuine difficulty squatting down to parallel or lower if these muscles can't carry out their responsibility appropriately.

One approach to strengthen the psoas is by doing the kind of toe-lifting movements I referenced toward the beginning of the article. However, for this position, I want to depend on closed-chain developments, where the hands are fixed and can't move. This little change makes it harder to cheat or compensate for, enabling you to concentrate squarely on the movement.

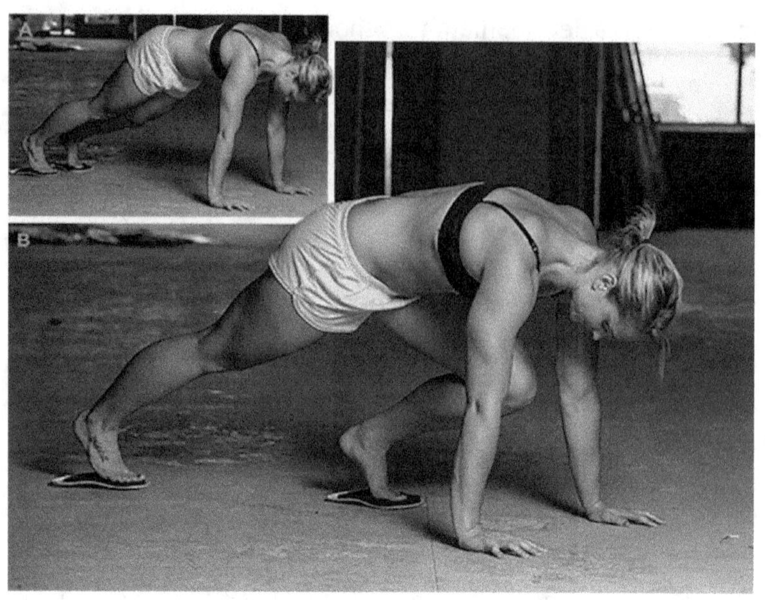

My exercise of choice here is floor-slide mountain climbers. You will need some furniture moving cushions, Valslides, or something comparable that will slide easily on your floor. Paper plates even function admirably when there's no other option. Put your feet on the sliders and move into a push-up position. To do the movement, force each knee, in turn, up toward your chest, going as high as you can while keeping your foot on the slider. You can alternate legs with every rep or do sets of each leg in turn. Try not to expect that it will be simple.

Floor Slides

Your hips may not lie, yet they can sidetrack your training if they drop askew. Put in place this three-section plan, and your hips will be progressively more powerful in the gym and less prone to injury moving forward!

In case you're keen on building hip quality that matters, however not keen on experiencing the outrage of the leg-spreading machines, you, fortunately, have other and better options.

Why You Need To Get Hip

The hip abductors and adductors are viewed as an antagonistic pair: As one muscle group gets, the other gathering relaxes. The abductors, including the gluteus medius, gluteus minimus, tensor fasciae latae, sartorius, and piriformis, are responsible for moving your leg away from your body's midline.

Generally, every time you make a lateral step or swing your leg off the side of the bed, your abductors are contracting. The adductors, fundamentally the adductor Magnus, minimus, brevis, and longus (with the gracilis and pectineus having an impact), do the contrary job, contracting at whatever point you have to draw your leg toward your body's midline.

The abductors specifically are notoriously weak in many individuals, which can add to back pain, among other issues. Weak adductors are an infamous supporter of both crotch strains and knee pain. So indeed, they matter. Presently here's the way to prepare them.

Wide-Stance Squat below Parallel

Each leg exercise should incorporate a squat variety. This closed-chain, compound development targets pretty much everything in your lower body, including your internal and external thighs. Be that as it may, to truly hammer your hips, you should be diving deep and turning your toes out.

Joshua Kruvand, the author and proprietor of Kru Strength + Fitness, directs explicitly toward a recent report that evaluated the squat depth and external hip pivot. The objective of the investigation was to examine the enrollment of the abductor bunch during a squat.

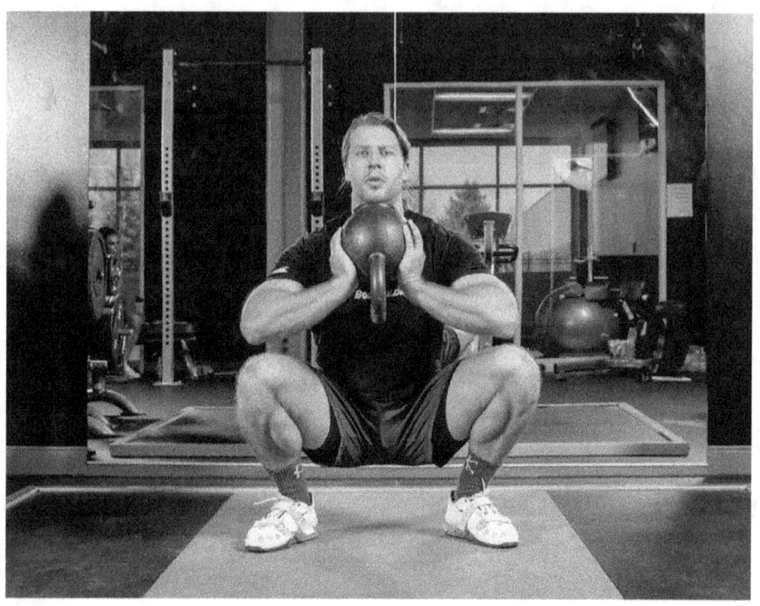

Scientists found that squats at or beneath parallel, and those with at any rate a 30-degree outer revolution of the hips (accomplished by calculating the toes slightly outward), were greatly improved when focusing on the abductor bunch rather than those with less knee flexion or interior hip rotation.

I don't get this meaning for you? Probably a portion of your squats should resemble this:

1. Stand tall with your feet generally at or marginally more extensive than shoulder-width apart. Edge your toes outward at somewhere in the range of 30 and 50 degrees. Connect with your center and check your stance, ensuring your shoulders are back and your chest is up.

2. Press your hips back and bring down your glutes toward the ground, keeping your weight in your heels. As you twist your knees, you'll need to draw in your abductor groups to keep your knees lined up with your toes.

3. When your hips dip under 90-degrees, stop, and at that point switch the movement by squeezing through your heels, broadening your knees and hips, and coming back to standing.

You can do this exercise with or without included weight, for example, hand weights, free weights, or portable weights. More significant than the method you choose is that you keep up maintain structure, with your knees following your toes.

Sumo Deadlift
The sumo deadlift uses a comparable foot position as the wide-legged squat, and it's this outside revolution of the hips that prompts the upgraded commitment of the internal and external thighs.

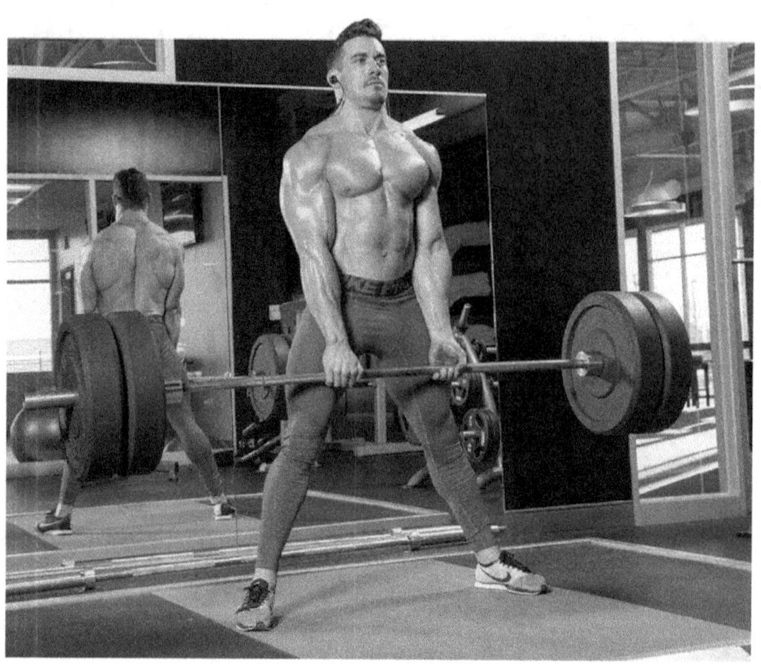

"When contrasted with a traditional deadlift, the sumo takes into consideration greater recruitment of the adductors and an additionally balancing out emphasis for the abductors," says Lindsey Cormack, an aggressive power lifter and CrossFit coach. "Doing sumo may feel less steady from the start, however, the balance requirement is the thing that enables you to adequately prepare both the abductors and adductors."

1. Stand behind a stacked free weight, situating your feet wide, with your toes calculated outward. Draw in your center and roll your shoulders back to guarantee you have a great stance. Then again, you can use an iron weight or a free weight on its side.

2. Press your hips back and lean forward, arriving with your arms straight down to get a handle on the weight. Curve your knees and lower your glutes toward the ground.

3. Take a full breath in, and, on your breathe out, pass through your heels, expanding your knees and hips couple as you come back to standing. Press your hips forward at the highest point of the movement, drawing your shoulder bones together and driving your chest forward.

4. Reverse the development in a controlled manner, squeezing your hips back before twisting your knees and bringing down your glutes toward the ground.

If you haven't done many of these, you will be sore down south for some time after your first exercise. Think about that as a sign that your hips required some attention.

Side-Lying Hip Abduction

A recent report, distributed in the Journal of Orthopedic and Sports Physical Therapy, found that the non-weight-bearing, side-lying hip abduction was as compelling at recruiting the gluteus medius (one of the essential hip abductors) as other, weight-bearing exercises.

You may think you don't have to take a physical-therapy-based approach to your hips. However, you may not be right. Genuinely weak hip muscles need disconnected consideration, not simply the pounding that overwhelming squats and sumo deadlifts can inflict.

The way that you needn't bother with loads for this exercise makes it an incredible isolation movement. Dr Alice Holland, of Stride Strong Physical Therapy, focuses on the side-lying hip grabbing as one of her top choices. She noticed that sprinters and athletes frequently battle with it, which means they need it more than anybody.

1. Lie on your side with your hips stacked over one another. Position your top leg behind your front leg by around 5 degrees, so your top heel is behind you.

2. Keeping your center drew in and your knee straight, lift your top lower leg toward the roof without moving your pelvis at all. Arrange yourself with your hands or elbows contrasting.

3. Return your top foot to the beginning position and keep up a gradual pace, and great, controlled form.

Side-Lying Hip Adduction

In logical electromyography testing, the side-lying hip adduction includes five different exercises (counting sumo squats and side jumps) for initiation of the adductor longus muscle.

Like its snatching partner, the adduction exercise can be done anyplace since you needn't bother with anything to do it except a comfortable mat. This makes it an incredible move to add to your center everyday practice or after squeezing in a quick home workout.

1. Lie on your side on the floor with your hips stacked vertically, one over the other. Connect with your center and prepare yourself, using your hands or elbows alternating. Ensure your hips stay fixed and opposite to the floor.

2. Keeping your middle and hips unyielding, twist your top knee and draw your foot toward your hips, planting it before your base leg.

3. Engage the adductors of your lower leg and lift your leg as high off the floor as you can without turning or tilting your pelvis (presumably just a

couple of inches). Hold for a second at the highest point of the movement, at that point gradually bring down your leg back to the beginning position.

If backs pain, knee pain, or SI joint pain are a part of your life, check out these developments. Remember about your hips! If you do, they might choose to remind you why they're significant all things considered.

Before we talk hip flexor stretches, we should take a look at the hip flexor itself.

These are the principle parts:

- Iliopsoas (the iliacus and psoas muscles)
- Sartorius
- Rectus femoris

The iliacus attaches on the upper part of the femur and starts within the peak of the ilium (within the pelvis), where the psoas joins completely through the transverse procedures of the lumbar spine, in any event, authoritative into the plates directly. The rectus femoris starts at the base of the front prevalent iliac spine, and attaches right down to the knee top, though the sartorius begins in a similar spot as the rectus femoris, yet connects on the average part of the knee, mixing with the MCL and parts of the hamstrings.

At the point when these muscles contract together without the use of the floor, we see hip flexion, as on account of a hanging leg raise. At the point when we see the muscles contract while the feet are reaching the ground, we see a variety of hip flexion known as front pelvic tilt.

The iliopsoas has an underrated role in spinal adjustment. It bodes well when you perceive how the psoas connects up and down the lumbar spine, giving pressure and adjustment against uncontrolled spinal flexion, sidelong flexion, and shear. It's a serious deal that way.

Interestingly enough, the psoas also has massively significant facial systems, with the average arcuate tendon giving a continuation directly to the stomach. Its lower fibers directly join to the pelvic floor. It's another motivation behind why breathing examples can affect everything.

So is the hip flexor tight in light of the fact that it's short, or in light of the fact that it's reacting to a feeble center?

It's regularly center brokenness. However, a weak core isn't just a failure to do crunches and stuff like that. It's the failure of the spine to keep up a steady and powerful foundation in a neutral pelvic position, with fabulously magnificent glute activation to drive the body forward.

One approach to effectively "stretch" the hip flexors is to get the pelvis balanced, or even into a back tilt while firing the living daylights out of your glutes. I'm not just discussing maximal intentional withdrawal. I'm talking cracking walnuts with your cheeks. The sort of weight that transforms a huge amount of coal into three carats of jewels or by making somebody hate their whole presence through a back foot-raised split squat concentrating on the vertical spine and pelvic tilt. (Well that is a hip flexor stretch!)

These will, in general, make individuals incapable of walking for a couple of moments in the wake of finishing them, particularly when they get into the right position where those hip flexors (especially the rectus femoris) stretch as far as possible under the burden.

If stretching these suckers doesn't create the ideal stretching of the hip flexors, we can deal with getting the center firm and stable, with the objective of abandoning the need for the iliopsoas to provide spinal stabilization. We can board the hell out of that sucker as long as we keep a balanced pelvis and spinal position.

In addition to planks, you can use hostile to growth, flexion, and turn exercises, which train the body to oppose outside difficulties to center stability.

You'll finish with hip expansion movements, during which the glutes act as an agonist to the hip flexors, and provide low back stability. By helping the center muscles settle the spine, they lessen the push on the psoas, hence diminishing the "tightness."

Glute stimulation to battle hip flexor stiffness is best with full-stretch expansion exercises like deadlifts and hip extensions. Fight the temptation to use, and then drop, massive amounts of weight while making loud grunting noises... Truly, it signals to everybody how amazing your customer is, yet it's not the prescribed method to lessen tight hip flexors.

"Why do I have lower back pain?"

Before you jump into the best exercises for lower back pain, it's important to understand that there are a large number of reasons why an individual could experience muscle soreness. On account of this article, we'll center on the most widely recognized one: sitting. After some time, prolonged sitting times can control our stance, causing specific muscles to become more fragile.

The established position anatomically implies we don't connect with our abs and glutes, which can cause them to turn off and fall asleep. The drop out of this is other muscles need to work more enthusiastically to compensate and support the body. The muscles in our lower backs become exhausted while our hip flexor muscles, for the most part, the psoas that attaches to the femur and lumbar spine become tight and tense. It's this unevenness that triggers the pain, particularly in our lower back.

3 Stretches to do for lower back pain

A typical offender in lower back pain due to sitting are tight or shortened hip flexors, which interface with your iliopsoas muscle, and regularly bring about weak or alternating lower back and glute muscles. The following compelling static stretches will help stretch out those muscles and convey lower back help. The ordinary act of these stretches will also help in improving your posture long-term.

Deep lunge stretch for hip flexors

Muscle stretched: Hip flexor

Count: 20 seconds on each side (hold for more as desired)

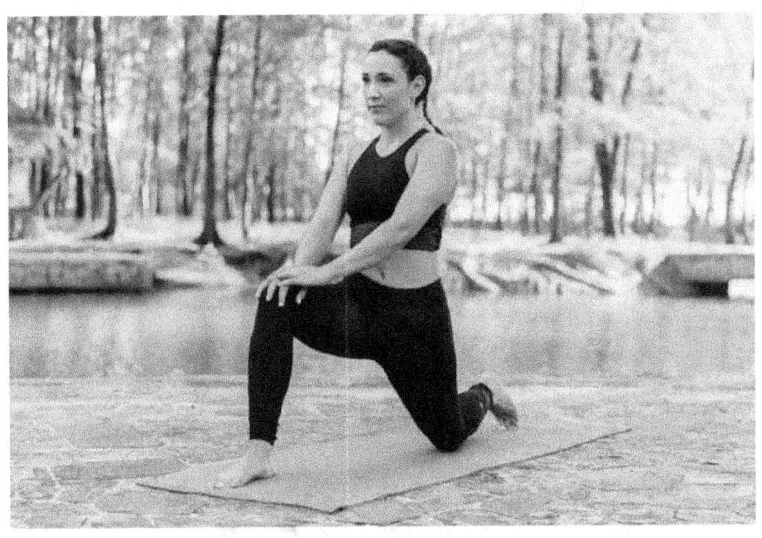

Step by step instructions to do one repetition:

1. Start on your knees, lean forward and place your hands on the floor/facing directly before you.

2. Place your right foot by your right hand alongside the thumb then, lift your hands off the floor, and place them on your hips for stability.

3. Raise your chest gradually until your middle is upright.

4. The right knee should be bowed at a 90° edge and directly over your right lower leg.

5. While breathing out, twist your right knee gradually and keep up an upright chest area.

6. Hold for 20 seconds. The stretch should be felt in the upper right thigh.

7. While breathing in, gradually recline to the start position.

8. Switch your leading leg and repeat.

Pigeon stretch to open hips

Muscle stretched: Hip flexor

Check: 20 seconds on each side (hold for more as desired)

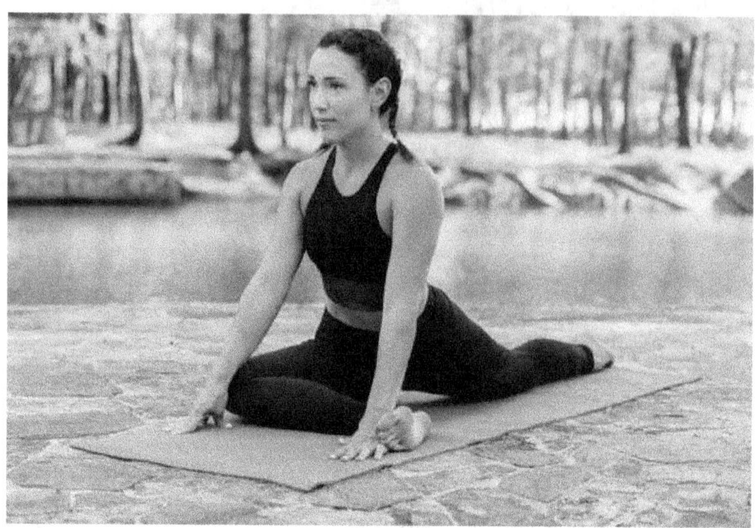

The most effective method to do one repetition:

1. Start on hands and knees with your arms shoulder-width and legs hip-width apart.

2. Place right knee forward behind the right hand. Place right lower leg as near to your left hip as conceivable without straining.

3. The right leg should lie directly on the floor with the right lower leg as near the left hand as could reasonably be expected. Depending upon your characteristic manageability, the more parallel the leg is with the front of the face, the more exceptional the hip opener.

4. Slide left leg back, fix and point toes directly behind your body with hips square.

5. Exhale and walk your fingertips forward, gently lowering the upper body down (place a pad or yoga mat under your butt.

6. Hold the stretch for 20 seconds and lay on your fingertips, lower arms or if OK with forehead on the floor.

7. Release the stretch gradually and turn around the movement by gradually lifting the chest and walking the hands back, raising the hips and go to start position for each of the fours.

8. Switch driving leg and repeat.

Cat-cow stretch to mobilize and release the spine
Muscles stretched: Spine

Check: Repeat 10-20 times

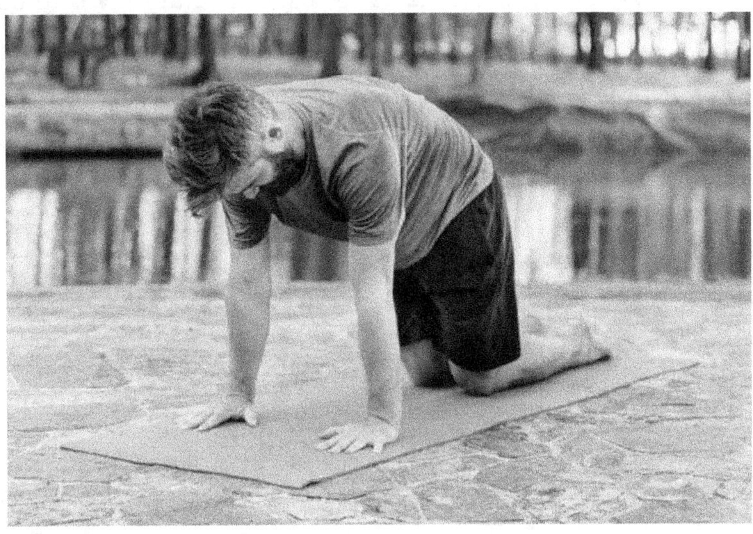

The most effective method to do one repetition:

1. Start on hands and knees with arms shoulder-width and legs hip-width apart.

2. Spread fingers easily wide for stability.

3. Your back should be in a tabletop position with head held neutral and looking downward.

4. Begin with: cow pose - Inhale and gradually direct your stomach towards the face and as you lift your jaw and chest simultaneously, look upwards.

5. Pull shoulders from the ears and hold for a second.

6. Transition directly into feline posture: Exhale and crush your tummy to your spine, adjusting your back with your head and jawline tucked into your chest, but don't force your jaw to your chest.

7. Hold for a second or two then change back to cow pose.

8. Repeat several times.

What are the best exercises for lower back pain?

There is no single best exercise for lower back pain; the key is to develop quality in your center and glutes, which regularly will, in general, be weak; consequently, the lower back stays at work longer than required to compensate. Strengthen your center and calm your lower back. The following are a choice of the best center and abdominal muscle exercises that don't strain your back directly from the 8 fit app.

Hyperextensions
Muscles included: Shoulders, lower back, abs, and glutes

Check: Count one each time you come back to start position

Tips:
- Keep shoulders back and down away from ears
- Keep chin down, neck neutral

Step by step instructions to do one repetition:

1. Lie face down on your stomach with hands at your sides and palms facing down.

2. Keep your hips and feet secured, at that point, lift your chest and hands off the floor.

3. Pause at the top, at that point, bring your chest and hands down to the floor.

Swimmers

Muscles included: Lower back, abs, glutes, and shoulders

Tally: Left-directly as one

Step by step instructions to do one repetition:

1. Lie face down on your stomach with arms loosened up straight in front and palms on the floor.

2. Lift your hands and feet off the floor until your body forms a curve from fingers to toes.

3. Simultaneously lift the left hand and the right foot higher, as your right hand and left foot drop lower.

4. Alternate sides and repeat movement. Every 2 kicks is considered 1 rep.

Tips:
*   Keep arms and legs straight, shoulders down away from ears
*   Keep chin down, neck neutral
*   Glute bridge

Muscles included: Glutes, hamstrings, lower back, and abs

Tally: Count one each time you come back to start position

The most effective method to do one rep:

1. Lie on your back with knees bowed and the bottoms of your feet on the floor.
2. Press your weight into your heels to raise your hips.
3. Lift your hips until your body form a straight line from shoulders to hips to knees, and press your glutes at the top.
4. Lower your hips down to come back to start position.

Tips:

- Keep core engaged for balance
- Press shoulder bones back and down to the floor
- Press hands into the floor for additional help

Plank Spiderman
Muscles included: Abs, shoulders, glutes, and triceps

Check: Left-directly as one

The most effective method to do one repetition:

1. Place elbows on the floor directly underneath your shoulders with lower arms parallel, legs straight behind, feet together and toes twisted under.
2. Tense each muscle to keep your body in a straight line from the head to heels.

3. Bring your right knee forward towards your right elbow, at that point come back to start position.

4. Repeat and bring your left knee toward your left elbow.

Tips:

- Keep the neck long, shoulders back and down away from ears
- Don't sink into shoulders
- Keep hips still and body in a straight line
- Breathe gradually and consistently, don't hold your breath

Air Plunge

Muscles included: Shoulders, back, chest

Tally: One each time you come back to start position

Step by step instructions to do one repetition:

1. Lie on your back with hands reached out at your sides, lower back squeezed onto the floor.

2. Bring your knees to your chest and kick straight legs up to lift hips from the floor.

3. Tuck your knees in towards your stomach and stretch out your legs directly to glide your feet a couple of steps off the floor.

4. Tuck your knees back to start position.

Tips:

- Keep the neck long with shoulders back and down away from ears
- Engage center and press lower bottom over into the floor

- For extra help, place hands under butt

Modified Plank

Muscles included: Shoulders, abs, triceps, hamstrings, and glutes

Check: 20-30 second hold

The most effective method to do one rep:

1. Sit on a mat; legs stretched out with your heels on the floor.
2. Place your hands directly under your shoulders.
3. Lean back on your hands and raise your hips off the floor.
4. Tense each muscle in the body to shape a straight line from your head to your heels.
5. Hold the position for the shown measure of time.

Tips:

- Keep the neck long, shoulders back and down away from ears
- Don't sink into the shoulders
- Keep center drawn in, hips up and body in a straight line
- Breathe gradually, don't hold the breath

Need to continue training from the comfort of home? Try some of our most loved at-home exercises.

Pain-free and stronger

To guarantee you have recognizable alleviation of lower back pain, focus on strengthening your center and loosening up exhausted muscles. This will also do wonders for posture and general prosperity. The sooner you include the above stretches and exercises to your everyday exercise schedule, the sooner your body will receive the rewards.

In case you're an exercise novice, the 8 fit exercises are also an incredible spot to begin as they are full-body exercises to reinforce and tone up, for a fitter you. I would urge you turn out, at least, four times each week, so you feel more grounded and can free yourself of lower back pain.

5 Exercises to Strengthen Your Hip Flexors

I bet you thought you'd see a lot of crazy exercises to strengthen your hip flexors, isn't that right?

Luckily, you don't have to do anything odd or insane or even purchase any weird fitness gadgets.

A considerable amount of the best exercises that train the muscles of the lower body additionally help fortify and activate the hip flexors.

Here are 5 of our strengthening exercises to reinforce your hip flexors:

Squat

Squats are the king of exercises, period.

They work a huge amount of muscles in the body (counting the hip flexors).

Essentially, in case you're not doing some hunching down example in your training program, you're passing up building more grounded glutes and firmer legs.

Presently, in case you're not open to hunching down with a free weight on your back, you can try any of these other squat varieties, including:

- Goblet Squats
- Split Squats
- Front Squats
- Landmine Squats
- Hack Squats
- Dumbbell squats
- Kettlebell squats

Bulgarian Split Squat

The greater, badder and crueler advance sibling of the conventional squat is the Bulgarian Split Squat.

What makes the Bulgarian Split Squat so devious?

You're doing a one-legged squat.

When doing the Bulgarian (or back foot raised) split squat, one leg is put on a crate, seat, or split squat stand while the other leg stays in contact with the ground and needs to do all the work.

After finishing all reps on one side, enjoy a short reprieve (30-60 seconds) and repeat on the opposite side.

Walking Lunge

Compared with the initial two exercises on this list, the rush is more powerful and complex as you need to step forward while delivering a pile and keep up an upright stance. In that capacity, the lunge is an incredibly athletic movement that enables working the muscles, provides quality, and stability in the muscles of the lower body, just like the hip flexors.

In case you're new to lunging, it's ideal, to start with just bodyweight lunges and when you feel great taking care of your bodyweight, progress to holding hand weights or portable weights and at last stir your way up to free weights.

Reverse Lunge

Not exclusively can lunges be done by stepping forward, yet they can likewise be done by taking a step in reverse.

Favorable circumstances of the turnaround jump are that it imposes the glutes and hamstrings more than the conventional strolling thrust and takes into account an incredible stretch of the hip flexors, an exceptionally welcome reward for those of us who battle with tight hips or possibly hip flexors.

At long last, the turnaround jump might be more reasonable for the individuals who manage knee pain during walking lunges. The explanation behind this is in a reverse jump; you're stepping in reverse and keeping an increasingly vertical shin point on the working leg, the two of which help lessen shearing muscles on the knee joint.

Band-Resisted Knee Drive

In conclusion, we have a more "isolation," a type of exercise for the hip flexors that likewise encourages you to chip away at creating energy in the band-opposed knee drive.

Loop a resistance band around a section, solid object, or use a door anchor attachment at the lower leg level.

Stand facing away from the anchor point with the band around your right lower leg. Push your right knee up until your thigh is at least parallel to the floor. Hold for a tally of one and afterwards gradually bring down your leg back to the ground.

Static Stretches to Improve Overall Hip Mobility and Flexibility

Hip Flexor Stretch
1. Kneel on your left side knee and put your right foot in front of you. Your right hip and knee should generally make a 90º angle. If this hurts your knee, don't hesitate to put a pillow under it.
2. Put your left hand to your left side hip and step by step, drive your hip forward. Your left hip should wind up before your left knee.
3. Make sure you keep your chest up and that you don't twist forward at the hips.

Hip Rotator Stretch
The hip rotators are significantly more functional than one may expect. The capability to turn the pelvis on the weight-bearing thigh. Hip rotators are used

in exercises, for example, swinging a golf club, moving, running, and tennis, yet they additionally do during basic exercises like walking.

Internal Rotators

This stretch should be done while sitting in a seat.

1. Cross your left leg over the right. Your left lower leg should lay over your right thigh.
2. Using your left hand, gently push down to your left side thigh until you start to feel opposition.
3. Tilt forward at the hips. Ensure your chest is up and your back is straight.
4. Hold this position for around 30 seconds, at that point, repeat on the opposite side.

External Rotators

This exercise should be done while sitting in a seat.

1. Cross your left leg over the right, so the left lower leg sits just past the right thigh.
2. Grab your left knee with two hands and put it back and to one side. If it helps, think about it as if you were pulling your knee towards your right shoulder.
3. Tilt forward at the hips gradually. Ensure your chest is up, your back is straight, and verify you aren't slouching.
4. Hold this position for 30 seconds.

Lying Hip Rotations

1. Lie on your back with the two knees bent upward and the two feet level on the ground.

2. Lift one foot and put it over the opposite knee.

3. Swivel your knee to and fro, keeping your lower leg on your opposite knee and your other foot level on the ground. Remember that only your twisted leg will be moving in this stretch.

4. Repeat for the opposite leg.

Standing Piriformis Stretch

1. While remaining with your back against a divider, walk your feet forward around 2 feet from the divider. At that point, bring down your hips at a 45-degree edge towards the floor.

2. Lift your right foot and put it over your left knee. The outside of your right lower leg should be opposite your left knee. You should feel a stretch in your glutes.

3. Hold for around 30 seconds, and at that point switch legs.

Butterfly Stretch

1. Sit on the floor and set up your feet together with the goal that your feet are pressed against each other.

2. Grab hold of your feet with two hands and press them into the ground. Simultaneously, twist at the hips to bring your crotch closer to your heels.

3. Hold for 30 seconds.

Travelling Butterfly

1. Sit on the floor with your back straight and your legs stretched straight before you.

2. Place your hands on the floor, somewhat behind your hips.

3. Use your hands to press into the ground and at the same time, lift your hips off the ground and advance towards your heels. You will end up in the butterfly position with your arms supporting your weight.

4. Return to the beginning position and repeat the stretch multiple times.

Hamstring Stretch

Sagittal Plane

1. Prop your decisive advantage over a seat or seat, making a point to keep it completely stretched.

2. While keeping your center tight, lean forward marginally until you feel a stretch in your hamstrings.

3. Hold this position for 30 seconds.

Transverse Plane

This stretch is equivalent to the sagittal plane stretch, then again, actually, you turn your leg from side to side once you have inclined forward. You should feel an alternate part of your hamstring stretch as your leg turns from within to the outside.

Hip Adductor Stretch

1. Assume lunge position by bowing to your left side knee and putting your right foot in front of you.
2. Slide your right foot out to the side and put two hands on the floor to balance yourself.
3. Keep your right knee straight and fit your body forward, keeping your hips loosened up at the same time.
4. Hold for 30 seconds, at that point repeat on the inverse side.

Leg Swings

1. Stand upright while clutching a seat, counter, or something of a comparable size for balance, trying to keep your feet pointed forward.
2. Bring your left leg before your right one, at that point expand your other leg until it is almost parallel with the floor. Ensure this is a smooth movement, and be certain not to kick.
3. Repeat multiple times and then switch sides.

Supine Hip Rotation

1. Lie down on your back with your knees bent and your heels on the floor.
2. Rotate your feet and knees out towards the floor, at that point pointing in towards one another.
3. Repeat multiple times.

Dynamic Stretches/Exercises to Improve Hip Mobility and Strength

Turn around Active Straight Leg Raise

1. Lie down on your back and bring your legs up, keeping them straight. Your back and legs should make as near a 90º angle as possible.
2. Using a tie or band, keep one leg straight up while gradually bringing down the other to the floor. Keep your center tight during this procedure since that is the thing that settles the spine and pelvis.
3. Repeat multiple times on each leg.

Single-Leg Hip Lift

1. Lie down on your back with the two feet fixed level on the floor. Your knees and calves should generally make a 90º angle.
2. Raise your right leg up straight with the goal that only your left foot is contacting the floor.
3. Using your glute muscles, bring your back up off the ground while keeping your head and shoulders firmly planted.
4. While loosening up the glutes, gradually bring down the butt and back towards the ground once more. Repeat multiple times, at that point, switch legs.

The Psoas of March

1. While lying level on your back, put your knees and feet together. At that point, bring them up off the ground so just your glutes, back, shoulders, and head are contacting the floor.
2. Slip an opposition band around the two feet.
3. Take turns stretching out each leg until it is straight. Repeat multiple times for each leg.

The Goblet Squat

1. Pick up a free weight or kettlebell, so you are using your hands to hold it somewhat under your jawline.

2. Spread your legs to somewhat past shoulder width and, stopping at the hip, drop into a squat position.

3. Pause at the base of the squat, at that point, with a tight center, use the glutes and legs to bring your body back up to a standing position.

Quality Training for the Hip and Pelvis

While these stretches will improve your hip mobility, quality training is another brilliant method to improve mobility and lessen the opportunity of injury. Here are some quality exercises that will work the hip flexor muscles:

- Bridges

- Split Squat

- Lateral Squat

- 4-Way Mini Band

- X Band Walk

- 4-Way Cable Hip

- Lateral Lunges

- Rotational Lunges

- Lateral Step Up

- Rotational Step Up

Therapy exercises for specific disorders

Iliopsoas bursitis

A recovery program for the iliopsoas disorder with hip turn (to expand portability), strengthening (of the hip muscles) and stretching exercises is intending to improve pain and working of patients with this syndrome.

Initial two weeks of the program

The internal rotation hip strengthening exercise

The patient should be in a sitting position. A flexible obstruction tie is used to do this exercise. The patient is sitting on the table. The flexible obstruction tie is attached to the table leg 10 cm over the floor. The opposite side of the obstruction tie is attached around the foot of the patient's affected hip.

The patient does an inside turn. The patient should do three groups of 20 repetitions on both the affected and unaffected side. At the point when the quality test reveals the affected side is more fragile than the unaffected side, then the number of sets on the unaffected side should be reduced to two groups of 20 reps rather than three sets.

Patients can experience exhaustion in the posterolateral hip area when they are doing the internal hip rotation exercise. The interior rotation strengthening exercise should be done daily and only on the affected side for about fourteen days. Following two weeks, the exercises will change to incorporate an increasingly functional position for the hip joint.

The external rotation hip strengthening exercise.
The same position as inside revolution; however, now the patient does an outer pivot. The tie is used to balance the thigh to prevent sagittal and frontal plane hip movement. This exercise can be used for patellofemoral pain syndrome. The patient should do three groups of 20 repetitions on both the affected and unaffected side.

At the point when the quality test reveals the affected side is weaker than the unaffected side, then the number of sets of the unaffected side should be decreased to two groups of 20 repetitions rather than three sets. Patients can encounter weakness in the anteromedial hip district when they are doing the outside hip turn. Following two weeks of the strengthening program, we do another exercise for about fourteen days.

The side-lying abduction/external rotation exercise
The patient lies on the table on his/her side with the hip at around 45 degrees of flexion (the elastic opposition band covers the knees). The person grabs his upper leg. He gradually brings down his leg: now the hip abductors contract eccentrically. The patient should do this exercise three groups of 20 repetitions on the affected side and two groups of 20 repetitions on the unaffected side. The side-lying snatching exercise should be done every day for about fourteen days. The underlying inside and outside exercises in sitting positions should be kept during this phase at a recurrence of a few times each week. At the one month point: the last part of the strengthening system.

Weightbearing hip strengthening exercise

The patient stays against the divider on one leg. The patient bears his weight on the affected side and he/she does a progression of smaller than usual squats. The patient should keep up the outer pivot of the affected hip with the goal that the hip stays over the straight part of the foot/leg, which is bearing the weight. This exercise should be done a few times each week with three groups of 20 strengthening on the affected side and two groups of 20 strengthening on the unaffected side.

Stretching program

The patients need to stretch every day. The primary stretches are: stretching of the hip flexor, the quadriceps, the horizontal hip/piriformis and the hamstring muscles. The patients should do a greater number of stretches on the affected side than on the unaffected side. They need to repeat them as frequently as they can for the day. They should continue stretching their muscles as long as they're in pain.

Piriformis disorder

Hip muscle Strengthening exercises and development re-education. For its position report, Tonley et al. depicts an elective treatment approach for piriformis disorder. The intervention concentrated on useful exercises planned for strengthening the hip extensors, abductors and outside rotators, just as the revision of broken development designs. Regardless of positive results (full goals of low back pain, postponement of butt cheek and thigh pain) for this position report, care must be produced in building up the cause and results for a single patient. Further examination is expected to extrapolate the results to other patients with piriformis disorder. The patient in this article pursued exercise based recuperation multiple times over a 3-month duration. The exercises are separated into more than 3 stages.

Stage 1 (week 0-4): non-weight-bearing exercises to accentuate isolated muscle recruitment

1) Bridge with Thera-band obstruction

- Wrap Thera-band around the thighs only proximal to the knee.
- Supine position + flexion of the knees and hip
- Elevate the pelvis, while meanwhile grabbing and doing an outside pivot of the hips.
- It's critical to stay away from adduction and inner pivot while bringing down the hip.
- 3 sets of 15 reps

2) Clamshells with thera-band opposition

- Sidelying, flexion of hip and knee in 45°, holding feet together
- Raise knees and back + hip grabbing and outside turn
- Use Theraband as the opposition and do 3 groups of 15 reps without obstruction.
- 3 sets of 15 repetitions

Stage 2 (week 4-9): Weight-bearing strengthening exercises

1) Squat with Thera-band opposition

- Wrap Thera-band around the thighs only proximal to the knee.
- Execute a squat move to a dept. of 45° (later 75°) with back

- 3 sets of 15 repetitions

2) Side-step with Thera-band opposition

- Wrap Thera-band around the thighs only proximal to the knee
- Squat position, 45° hip and knee flexion
- Take steps to one side and the left along with a 10-m walk-away
- Keep trunk erect during the exercise
- Avoid placing the knees over the toes
- 3 sets of 15 repetitions

3) Single-limb sit to stand

- Sit on a treatment table (start at 70 cm)
- Squat position
- Stand up and control hip movements and keep the arrangement of lower furthest point in frontal and transverse planes during the exercise
- Progress by bringing down the surface in 4 cm increases, twofold limbed to single-limbed
- 3 sets of 15 repetitions

4) Step Down

- Stand on a 20 cm high advance stool
- Touch the heel to the ground and return gradually to the start position once again a 3-second time frame
- Control hip movements and keep the arrangement of lower furthest point in frontal and transverse planes during the descending and ascending

- Do with contralateral furthest point bolster first, later without help (if you can execute 3 groups of 15 repetitions with control of hip movements)

Stage 3 (week 9-14): Functional Training, in particular, unique and ballistic training

1) Forward lunge

- The lead knee is flexed to a dept. of 75°
- Don't pass the knee past the foot
- Keep alignment femur in frontal and transverse planes during the exercise
- 3 sets of 15 reps

2) Lateral Lunge at 45°

- The lead knee is flexed to a dept. of 75°
- Don't pass the knee past the foot
- Keep alignment femur in frontal and transverse planes during the exercise
- 3 sets of 15 repetitions

3) Double limb take-off jumps with double-limb landings

- Do maximal effort double-limb take –off jumps to double-limb landings to a deep squat, with flexion of the knee (90°), without hip adduction or inside turn
- Control hip movements and keep the arrangement of lower limit in frontal and transverse planes
- 3 sets of 15 repetitions

4) Double limb take-off jumps with single-limb landings

- Do maximal effort double-limb take –off jumps to single-limb arrivals, with flexion of the knee (90°), without hip adduction or internal revolution
- Control hip movements and keep the arrangement of lower furthest point in frontal and transverse planes
- 3 sets of 15 repetitions

Treatment exercises to improve a few capacities
Strength

- Pelvic drop

This is a simple exercise to improve the quality in the gluteal muscles. Via training these muscles, you will have the option to avoid hip issues, as well as back or knee issues. Also, you can keep up suitable and useful mobility.

Remain on a stage stool. Hang one leg off the edge and keep your abs tight and your pelvis level. Let this leg gradually fall towards the ground by enabling your pelvis to gradually drop down. Drop your pelvis down quite far (your foot may not contact the ground) and hold this position for two seconds. After these two seconds, raise your pelvis by using the hip muscles in your support leg. Repeat this exercise a couple of times (10-15). If it turns out to be anything but difficult to do, you can hold a dumbbell to make it harder. During the execution of this exercise, it's critical to keep straight and your abs tight. Your support leg should also stay straight.

Single-Leg Adductor and Abductor Stretches with Strap
What It Does: Stretches the hip's adductor (crotch and internal thigh) and abductor (gluteus medius, gluteus minimus, and tensor fasciae latae) muscles, just as the IT band, to improve the versatility of the hip joint.

The most effective method to Do It: Continuing from the last stretch, with your leg still raised, use the tie to delicately bring down your leg out to the side, opposite to your body, until you feel a stretch in the inward thigh and crotch area (the hip-adductor muscles). Lower your leg to the extent you can easily stop moving your pelvis. Like previously, the thought is to keep your pelvis level, square, and stable all through the stretch. Hold pressure for a moment, at that point, move the leg over your body the other way to focus on the hip abductor muscles and IT band. Hold this stretch for a moment too, at that point repeat with the other leg.

Single-Leg Circles: Advance the single-leg stretch by gradually moving your leg in bigger and bigger circles (using the band to control the movement) to investigate the end range of your hip portability. Keep your leg straight, and do five to ten circles a clockwise direction, at that point repeat the other way. Be careful about any clicking or hard stops, as that may be an indication of hip impingement. Concentrate on keeping your pelvis level, square, and stable all through the stretch.

Couch Stretch
What It Does: Stretches the hip flexors to improve augmentation of the hip joint.

The most effective method to Do It: Kneel on the ground, confronting endlessly from a divider. Place one knee in the corner where the floor and divider meet, with your shin running up toward the roof and parallel to the divider. Move your other foot out before you so its level on the floor, with your knee, twisted at 90 degrees. Raise your middle, and carefully rush forward to sink further into the stretch. Hold the stretch for one to two minutes for each side.

"The thought here is to keep the knee near the divider and get your middle as upright as conceivable without angling through the lower back," Kechijian says.

If that this position is excessively troublesome, attempt to do a similar stretch with your foot on a seat, a chair, or a sofa (something generally knee size) rather than in a bad spot. This variety is simpler for individuals who have extremely tight quads and hip flexors.

Agility

Hamstrings

This exercise is to stretch the hamstrings. You can use this with shortened or stiff hamstrings.

Straight leg raise test: The patient lays on his back before a divider. The hip is in a neutral position (the hip point can change). At that point, he/she puts his heel against the divider. The passive tension is applied by continuously expanding the hip flexion edge. The patient holds his leg, without moving, during 10 seconds noticeable all around against the divider. After the 10 seconds, the patient needs to bring his leg gradually to the floor.

The patient repeats this exercise 4 x 10 seconds. The patient needs to quit raising the leg when his pelvic pivots. It's a sort of compensation. The worth can be estimated with three instruments: goniometer, flexometer, and measuring tape. This exercise can also be executed as a passive exercise.

The patient needs to lay on a table. The hip should be expanded to 180°. Presently the specialist raises the leg from the patient, as high as possible. Duration: The specialist holds the leg noticeable all around for 10 seconds and repeats this multiple times.

Tonley JC et al, who had a substitute hypothesis about the reason for piriformis disorder (see etiology piriformis disorder), depicted an elective treatment approach for piriformis disorder. The patient in this article pursued non-intrusive treatment multiple times over a 3-month term. The program was focused on strengthening the hip extensors, abductors and outer rotators, as well as development re-teaching. The exercises were separated into more than 3 stages.

The primary stage (week 0-4) contained non-weight-bearing exercises to emphasise confined muscle enrollment. This stage included two exercises, in particular, 'connect with Thera–band obstruction' and 'calm with thera–band opposition'. The reciprocal scaffold was executed with the Thera-band folded over his thighs only proximal to the knee. The patient must lift his pelvis, with temporary freezing and external rotation of his hips. It's imperative to maintain a strategic distance from adduction and inner pivot while bringing down the hip.

The clam exercise was done by side-lying, first without obstruction. The purpose of deviation includes flexion of hip and knee at 45° angle while holding his feet together. At that point, the patient raises his knee up and back, which was developed by hip grabbing and an outer turn. Sooner or later, the Thera-Band was used as the opposition during exercise. On the condition, that the patient must have the option to do 3 groups of 15 repetitions of the exercise without opposition.

Stage 2 (week 4-9) contains weight – bearing strengthening exercises. The patient began at first with double-limb weight-bearing exercises. A short time later, the patient did single-limb developments to increase the requests on the hip musculature. This stage included four exercises. The main exercise was a squat move done with the Thera–band opposition, which was applied around the thighs only proximal to the knees. The squat was first executed to a depth of 45° and later on to 75 °.

During the second exercise, the patient did a sidestepping exercise with a Thera-Band. The patient started the exercise in a squat position of 45° of hip and knee flexion. In this manner, he made moves to one side, and the left along a 10-m walk-path by seizing and externally rotating his hips. It is significant to keep the trunk erect during exercise and to avoid putting the knees over the toes.

The following exercise, named single – limb sit to stand, was executed similar to the squat. The patient did the exercise first from a 70-cm (estimated from the floor to the highest point of a treatment table) high surface. When he could do 3 groups of 15 repetitions; the stature was each time decreased by 4 cm, to the last height of 58 cm.

The last exercise rang the progression/step-down exercise. The patient used a 20-cm-high advance stool. The exercise was done by contacting his heel to the ground and returning gradually to the start position once again a 3-second time span. First, the patient had contralateral upper point support. This support was evacuated when the patient had the option to control his hip movements and to do 3 groups of 15 repetitions.

Stage 3 (week 9-14) comprised of Functional Training, to be dynamic and ballistic preparing. This phase incorporates 4 exercises. The movement in this stage was accomplished by expanding the pace during the exercise.

At first, the patient does forward lurches (figure 6A) and later he advances to sidelong rushes (figure 6B), to one side and the right at a 45° angle. The lead knee is flexed to a profundity of 75 °. It's not allowed to pass the knee past the foot. At the point when the patient was able to do 3 groups of 15 reiterations, he advanced to the sidelong rushes.

The third exercise was twofold appendage take – off bounces with twofold appendage arrivals to a profound squat, with flexion of the knee (90°), without hip adduction or inside rotation(figure 6C). The fourth and last exercise included additionally the twofold appendage take-off hops, yet now right and left single-appendage arrivals. (Figure 6D) Excessive hip adduction or interior turn is still not permitted.

Supine Figure-Four Stretch
What It Does: Stretches the outer hip-rotator muscles (piriformis, prevalent and second rate gemellus, interior obturator, and quadratus femoris).

How to Do It: Lie on your back with your knees bowed. Lift your left leg and traverse the right with the goal that your left lower leg rests just below your right knee. Raise your right leg, grab your right thigh, and gently pull it toward your chest. Hold this stretch for one to two minutes, then repeat on the opposite side.

More Tips

- If your hips are strong, take additional consideration to heat up gradually before exercise.
- Always turn out or stretch after exercise to decrease the stiffness and inflammation caused by the exercise.
- Limit the amount of time you spend sitting in a seat. In case you're a workplace exerciser, set up a standing work area, sit on an exercise ball, or get up and move as frequently as possible.

5 Simple Exercises to Fix the Injury Your Desk Job Causes

We get down to business trusting our days spent at the workplace will challenge us expertly, yet as a general rule, living the 9-to-5 (or 6 or 7) workplace life can be requested on the wellbeing and health front, as well.

Truth be told, as indicated by the U.S. Authority of Labor Statistics, business-related musculoskeletal issues from muscle strains to carpal passage disorder made up 32% of all specialist injury and disease cases in 2014. Of course, a considerable lot of those injuries were suffered by individuals working construction lines or doing other physically taxing jobs. But, sitting hunched over a PC, writing irately and staring at screens throughout the day, can also wreak havoc on the body.

Generally, the blame lies unequivocally on what extent you sit while working at your work area. "The issue that we're truly facing is we're not made to sit—positively not for prolonged timeframes," says Michael Fredericson, sports drug physiatrist at Stanford Health Care. Anyway, when your office work calls for you to sit at a work area for quite a long time, "You will in general hunch forward, and your neck projects, and there's eye strain. It's pressure that affects your entire body."

The good news is that, along with doing some basic stretches, making ergonomic changes to your workplace can essentially decrease the daily distress most workers manage. And, the advantages go past the physical. A recent report found that developing more ergonomic workstations in the workplace decreased musculoskeletal and vision issues, yet, in addition, helped representatives' have more fulfilment and joy.

Obviously, at whatever point you're in pain, you should talk with your doctor to understand any fundamental issues or treatment concerns. However, with a part of the following moves and master tips, you could be en route to keeping the most infamous work area risks under control.

Work area JOB DANGER NO. 1: LOWER BACK PAIN
Regardless of whether it's an incidental twinge or a progressing ache, back pain can prevent you from doing your best. Sitting anchored to your work area for a considerable length of time can prompt lower back pain, the most widely recognized business-related issue.

So what precisely is going on back there? Drooping back in your work area seat or slumping forward means your spine is lopsided. That places a strain on the ligaments and muscles in your back.

The most effective method to Quickly Relieve Tension: To overcome muscle pressure when it crops up, rock your pelvis to and fro while positioned in your work area seat, tilting your hips up and adjusting your back, and then tilting your hips back. "That will help mend those tight muscles," says Stephen Aguilar, worldwide advisor and confirmed ergonomic appraisal expert at UCLA Rehabilitation Services.

The Long-Term Fix: Get some help. The length of your back should come to the rear of your seat to assist you with sitting upright. If there's a hole, use a lumbar pillow for cushioning to help keep yourself from falling forward or backward into a poor posture. Additionally, ensure your feet are laying level on the floor, with your thighs parallel to the ground.

"You need to keep from having your feet dangling off your seat," Aguilar says. "Something else, the heaviness of your leg isn't upheld, which puts more strain on your back." Using a hassock can help nix the discomfort.

Breaking a sweat can also help. The stomach exercises, for example, crunches, done a few times each week can strengthen your core. That eases the heat off your back and makes it simpler to keep up a great stance.

Work area JOB DANGER NO. 2: WRIST STRAIN

Going through your days and nights pounding away at your console, reacting to messages or writing reports can cause injuries that can turn into a genuine medical problem.

A mix of overuse and how you're positioning your wrists at your console are at fault. "At whatever point you work at a console or with a mouse, the tendons in your wrists go to and fro," Aguilar says. "These tendons are parallel to one another, so they float to and fro and make contact, which [is called] a micro trauma. That tedious movement causes weakness, and the tendons may get inflamed."

A less obvious factor that has a role in wrist pain: Poor stance, specifically having your shoulders hunched forward. That is because the position reduces the bloodstream downstream, including to your hands, causing soreness or at times, a tingling sensation or numbness.

Step by step instructions to Quickly Relieve Tension: Do a prayer stretch, otherwise called a Buddha stretch: Place your fingers and palms together with your hands before your chest, fingers facing upward. While keeping your palms together and your elbows moving out, bring down your hands until you feel a decent stretch in your wrists. Hold for five seconds.

The Long-Term Fix: When you're using the console or mouse, hold your wrists normally, so they're skimming on a level plane noticeable all around and not perched higher than your hands or laying around your work area. Additionally, get a wrist rest for your console and mouse, proposes Aguilar, and use it to take occasional breaks through the span of the day. "The catchphrase there is rest," he says.

Work area JOB DANGER NO. 3: NECK AND SHOULDER PAIN

You never acknowledge exactly the amount you move your neck and shoulders until they're injured, and afterwards, you feel every move and bend. These aches and pains may originate from putting your console or PC screen excessively far away around your work area, making you stick your neck and shoulders forward, throwing them forward and twisted with the spine and stressing the muscles and soft tissue.

Instructions to Quickly Relieve Tension: It might be tempting to pop two or three ibuprofen to dull the distress, however, a recent report found that successive neck and shoulder stretches regularly were more compelling at facilitating pain than over-the-counter and pain relieving drugs or in any event, seeing a chiropractor.

To release a tight neck, Fredericson suggests attempting a chin fold exercise, otherwise called neck withdrawal. While standing or sitting upright, keep your spine straight and drive your head forward, sticking your chin out beyond what many would consider possible. Gradually turn around the movement by pulling your head back beyond what many would consider possible, as though withdrawing ceaselessly from somebody. Your head should remain level all through the stretch, which you'll feel at the base of your neck. Repeat several times.

To relieve tension in your neck and shoulders all the while, look ahead, tilt your right ear down toward your right shoulder, leaving your left arm hanging straight down to build the stretch. Hold for 20 to 60 seconds and repeat on the other side several times.

The Long-Term Fix: Station the PC screen straightforwardly before you and not calculated to the side, which puts your neck into a bad position. In case you're on the telephone much of the time, use a headset as opposed to supporting the telephone between your ear and shoulder, which can cause muscle strain, says Jeffrey A. Goldstein, medicinal executive of NYU Langone Seaport Orthopedics. Use a seat with flexible armrests that enable your elbows to form a 90-degree angle. Aguilar clarifies that the armrest and the arm's angle help take the pressure off the shoulders.

"Great stance is also a more stretched time arrangement," he says. Take a stab at using an app that encourages you to chip away at improving your stance, as Posture Zone, which is free. In case you're extremely sincere about your endeavors, Lumo Lift ($79.99) uses a lightweight wearable sensor that vibrates when you're slouching and is an application that tracks your posture habits.

Work area JOB DANGER NO. 4: EYE STRAIN
Looking at your PC for quite a long time can cause eye fatigue, as can having a PC screen that is excessively far away (making your eyes strain to peruse the important part) or excessively close (making your eyes work more earnestly to center). Individuals also will, in general, squint less frequently while looking at their PC, which prompts dry eyes and fatigue.

The most effective method to Quickly Relieve Tension: Every 20 to 30 minutes, look at something far away, for example, a window while working, for 20 seconds to offer your eyes a break. Even better, get up and talk with a coworker in another area of the workplace or run to the stock storeroom to grab another pen, anything to offer your eyes a break from the PC.

The Long-Term Fix: The Occupational Safety and Health Administration prescribes guaranteeing that your PC screen is 20 to 40 inches from you, so it's not very close or excessively a long way from where you're sitting. The highest point of the PC screen should be generally at eye level. You can also put a barrier over your screen to lessen glare, which adds to eye strain.

If you wear glasses at work, do a ballpark estimation of the space between your eyes and the PC screen. At that point, check with your optometrist to ensure you have the right solution for that distance. "Numerous individuals wear glasses or contacts, however, they're intended for reading or distance," Aguilar says. "However, the PC is in the middle of the two distances. Get a solution for that PC distance and leave the pair at your office."

Work area JOB DANGER NO. 5: TIGHT HIPS

After some time, being stuck sitting in a twisted position every day from being at your work area to your sofa at home shortens your hip flexors, a group of muscles located at the front of your hips, causing pain. Tight hip flexors also add to causing back soreness, another basic objection.

Step by step instructions to Quickly Relieve Tension: Try doing a stretch to release tight hip flexors. Stoop to your left side knee, like you are going to propose to somebody and put your right foot forward with your right knee bent at a 90-degree angle. Move your pelvis forward, twist your front knee and fold your butt under until you feel a deeper stretch in the left hip. Hold for 30 seconds. Switch legs.

The Long-Term Fix: Stand up from your work area at ordinary intervals to offer your muscles a break and increase circulation. "Ideally, get up from your work area each 20 to 30 minutes," Aguilar says. "Your body needs to move."

Have a go at using a free application, for example, Stand Up! Or then again use Break Reminder which is an app that lets you set an alarm clock to remind you to get up at specific intervals through the course of the day.

By talking with your PCP and looking at a portion of these moves, you should have the option to assist yourself in feeling great at work or if nothing else make your body increasingly comfortable.

Quad and Hip Flexor Stretches and Exercises
Quad and hip flexor stretches are significant for the adaptability and scope of movement of the quadriceps (thigh) and iliopsoas muscles. Great quad and hip adaptability take into consideration unrestricted, pain-free development of the hip and upper leg.

Sports that Benefit from Quad and Hip Flexor Stretches

Sports that profit by the quad and hip flexor stretches below include: group exercises like netball, football, field, soccer, rugby and hockey. Also, any game that includes a great deal of running or walking, for example, track, cross country hiking, backpacking, mountaineering, orienteering and race walking.

Cycling, mountain biking, moving, artful dance, paddling, golf and combative techniques additionally help with the normal quad, and hip flexor stretch.

Quad and Hip Flexor Muscles being stretched

While doing the quad and hip flexor stretches below there are various muscles inside the hip and quads that are stretched. The following is a complete list of the anatomical muscle names engaged with the accompanying stretches.

- Psoas Major and Minor (Upper Hip);

- Iliacus (Upper Hip);

- Sartorius (Upper Quadriceps);

- Rectus Femoris (Upper Quadriceps; and

- Vastus Lateralis, Medialis and Intermedialis (Quadriceps).

Quad and Hip Flexor Stretching Safety Guidelines

Similarly, as with any game or action, there are rules to guarantee they are protected. Stretching is no special case. Stretching can be harmful and cause damage whenever done inaccurately. It is crucially significant that the following rules be adhered to, both for security and for boosting the advantages of the stretches.

- Breathe. Try not to hold your breath. Holding your breath causes strain and worry in your muscles, and can raise your circulatory strain. The deeper you inhale, the more loosened up your muscles will be, and the deeper and longer you will have the option to stretch.

- Never push a stretch past the purpose of gentle distress. Stretching tight muscles can be awkward, yet you should never feel any sharp or cutting pain. If you do, stop quickly; you are pushing the stretch excessively far.

- Be predictable. Stretching for a couple of moments two or three times each day will bit by bit build adaptability and range of movement over the long-term. This is a superior method of stretching, as opposed to stretching for a more drawn out time just once per week.

- Wear-comfy clothes, as it's hard to stretch if your garments are tight and limit movement.

Test Quad and Hip Flexor Stretches

Slowly move into the stretch position until you feel a strain of around 7 out of 10. If you feel pain or inconvenience you've pushed the stretch excessively far; pull out of the stretch right away. Hold the stretch position for 20 to 30 seconds while relaxing and breathing deeply. Leave the stretch cautiously and do the stretch on the opposite side if necessary. Repeat 2 or more times.

Standing Reach-up Hip Flexor Stretch: Stand upright and step forward. Reach up with two hands, drive your hips forward, lean back and then lean away from your back leg. Hold this stretch for around 20 to 30 seconds and repeat at least 2 or more times on each side.

Single Lean-back Quad Stretch: Sit on the ground, twist one knee and put that foot by your bum. At that point, gradually lean backward. As above, hold this stretch for around 20 to 30 seconds and repeat at least 2 or more times on each side.

Test Quad and Hip Flexor Stretching Videos

Below you'll see a couple of good stretches for your quads and hip flexors. However, don't depend on only a couple of stretches; it's important to do a range of stretches for the bum, hamstrings, hips, crotch and core. If you don't mind, be cautious, if you haven't stretched your quads and hip muscles, a portion of these stretches will put a great deal of weight on the muscles and ligaments. Warm-up first, then, continue in a gradual and gentle way.

If you would prefer not to walk around every single hunched shoulder and mix steps like an 80-year-old when you're 40, you have to make stretching a requirement. Ordinary stretching can help keep up and improve the range of movement and mobility, forestall injuries, and ease chronic pain, especially pain brought about by irregular muscle characteristics expedited by an excessive amount of sitting.

Also, stretching feels good. It resembles a relaxing, energizing rest for your entire body. And keeping in mind that there are several stretches to browse, in case you're searching for open, safe stretches that focus on each significant muscle groups, you can't turn out badly with the choices on this list.

Daniel Fishel/Thrillist
Triceps: Overhead triceps stretch

At times, the oldies are as yet the best. This triceps stretch goes back to primary school, and its effectiveness is still valid.

- Stand tall with great posture. Reach your left arm out of sight over your head, then twist your elbow, putting your left-hand level on your upper back, as adaptability permits.
- With your right hand, take your left arm, put it simply over the elbow, and use your right hand to lightly pull your left elbow toward your head as your left hand arrives at a more remote spot down your back. You should feel a stretch through your left triceps.
- When you feel a decent stretch, hold for 20 to 30 seconds before swapping sides.

Daniel Fishel/Thrillist

Biceps: Standing biceps stretch

The biceps muscles cross two joints, the shoulder and the elbow. To successfully stretch the biceps, you need to stretch every one of these joints. One great alternative is the standing biceps stretch, which is some of the time called the "chest opener," as it can also be used to stretch the chest and shoulders.

- Stand tall, feet shoulder-distance apart, knees somewhat bent. With your arms broadened, fasten your hands directly, palms touching.
- From this position, pivot your wrists in reverse, opening your still-clasped hands, so your palms are facing the floor.
- Keeping your elbows straight, raise your arms behind your body until you feel a stretch through your biceps. Hold for 20 to 30 seconds, release, and repeat. To get a deeper stretch through your shoulders and chest, turn upward toward the roof and draw your shoulders in reverse to broaden your chest.

Daniel Fishel/Thrillist

Lower arms: Alternating wrist pull

Lower arms kinda get the shaft in regard to stretching and strengthening, but if you do a ton of composing, they probably deserve a decent stretch.

- From a seated or standing position, stretch out the two arms sensibly before your chest. Flex your left wrist toward you, so your fingers point upward, then turn it to the outside until your fingers point toward the floor.

- Clasp your left palm with your right hand and gently pull your left hand toward you until you feel a stretch through your left lower arm. Hold for 10 seconds, then switch sides. Repeat a few times for each side.

Daniel Fishel/Thrillist

Shoulders: Cross-body shoulder stretch

Given that your shoulders are engaged with basically every chest area movement you do, that means they're associated with practically every chest area stretch you do, as well. The decent thing about the cross-body shoulder stretch is it focuses on the backside of your shoulder and into your upper back.

- Stand with your feet shoulder-width apart; knees marginally bowed, the two arms stretched out and down at your sides.
- Keeping your left elbow straight, raise your left arm legitimately before your chest, at that point put over your body, toward your right shoulder.
- Bend your right elbow and hold your left arm just beneath the elbow with your right hand. Use your right hand to gently press your left arm nearer to your chest. At the point when you feel a decent stretch through your shoulder and into your triceps, hold the position for 20 to 30 seconds before exchanging sides.

Daniel Fishel/Thrillist

Back: Cat, bovine, kid's pose movement

There are many, many muscle groups that range the length and broadness of your back. Also, in light of the fact that these muscles are engaged with such a large number of various movements at such huge numbers of joints, it's difficult to pick only one stretch that works admirably at keeping up mobility and managing stress.

- That is the reason I've picked a typical yoga-based grouping that truly works admirably at focusing on your whole back, while also stretching the chest, shoulders, abs, and hips. Besides, the feline, bovine exercise is known to help mitigate low-back pain, a very basic plague of present-day life.

- Start on your hands and knees on an exercise mat, your palms situated under your shoulders, your knees situated under your hips, and your back and neck in a flat (neutral) position.

- Enter cow pose as you breathe in by looking upward and stretching your chest forward as you are pressing your hips upward, attempting to express your tailbone toward the roof. This exercise will cause your low back to plunge toward the floor, stretching your abs all the while. Hold for a count of three.

- Enter the feline posture as you breathe out by bringing down your head between your shoulders and tucking your tailbone under, scooping your hips forward and squeezing your upper back and shoulders toward the roof. Round your shoulders outward to widen the stretch over your upper back. Use your abs to keep your hips scooped forward to feel a pleasant stretch through your low back and hips. Hold for a count of three.

- Return to a neutral, tabletop-like position on your next breath in, at that point as you breathe out, enter the kid's posture by sitting out of sorts, your chest folding over your quads as you put out your arms the extent that you can over your head, your palms level on the ground. Hold this position for three full breaths, truly sinking your hips into your heels with each breath out.

- After three breaths, come back to the tabletop position and do three to five additional rounds of the group.

Chest: Wall-helped single-arm chest stretch

- A portion of different exercises on this list have just helped loosen up the chest, yet to truly focus on each side of your body, you can't go wrong with the divider assisted single-arm chest stretch.
- Stand with your left side opposite to a divider, around 1 to 2 ft away from the divider.
- Reach your left arm behind you, your elbow stretched, and place your left palm level on the divider. Start with your hand situated, so your left arm is parallel to the floor.
- You should feel a stretch through your chest and the front of your shoulder. To develop the stretch, move your weight toward the divider, or gradually draw your feet nearer to the divider. At the point when you feel a decent stretch, hold the position for 20 to 30 seconds before exchanging sides.
- You can change the edge of the stretch by situating your palm higher or lower on the divider.

Daniel Fishel/Thrillist

Abs: Stability ball-helped backbend

Backbends are an incredible method to stretch the whole front part of your body, from your chest and shoulders, down your core and into your hip flexors and quads. Unfortunately, the vast majority of those older than 25 have some hard memories of using their bodies like an Olympic gymnast.

Enter: The stability ball. Pretty much anybody can do an incredible stomach muscle, hip, chest, and shoulder stretch by doing a changed backbend using a stability ball for help.

- Sit on a stability ball; your feet fixed shoulder-width apart and your knees bent at 90-degree angles.
- Slowly step forward as you at the same time recline, resting over the ball.
- With your knees still bowed, extend your arms over your head and put them backward, permitting your back to curve with the help of the ball. You should feel a decent stretch through your abs, chest, and shoulders.
- Continue going backward to the extent that you can, and if you feel good, advance your feet forward, stretching out your knees to get a stretch through your quads and hip flexors.
- Hold the supported backbend for 30 to 60 seconds, breathing deeply all through it.

Daniel Fishel/Thrillist

Glutes: Supine figure-4 glute stretch

In case you're active, especially in case you're a sprinter who ignores broadly educating, nothing feels on a par with a deep glute stretch. The muscles of the glutes, especially those associated with hip grabbing, the gluteus medius and minimus - are inclined to be disregarded. They're regularly not strengthened as much as a percentage of different muscles of the lower body, and they're inclined to lengthening and weakening in people who do a great deal of sitting.

These combined effects lead to a wide range of uneven muscles in the glutes, low back, and hips, which a decent glute stretch can help resolve.

- Lie on your back, your knees twisted, and feet level on the floor. Crisscross your left knee, as though making a "4" with your legs.
- Contract your abs to hold your low back in contact with the ground, then lift your left foot from the floor. Place the two arms forward to get ahold of the rear of your left thigh.
- From this position, use your arms to pull your left leg closer to your body to stretch it out. Keep your right knee indicated on the side of the room - don't let it adduct toward your midline. In case you're adaptable enough, you can use your right elbow to press your right knee away. At the point when you feel a profound stretch through your right glute, hold the position for 20 to 30 seconds before exchanging sides.

Daniel Fishel/Thrillist

Quads: Standing quad stretch

- You're likely acquainted with the standing quad stretch, another physed top pick. There's no motivation to upset something worth being thankful for.
- Stand tall, feet fixed generally hip-separation apart, knees somewhat bent.
- Shift your weight to one side's foot, twist your right knee behind you, and lift your right foot toward on the other side's glute.
- Grasp the highest point of your right foot with your right hand to crush your right impact point nearer to your glute. Ensure your right knee is touching the ground, your right leg is still lined up with your left leg. At

the point when you feel a decent stretch, hold the position for 20 to 30 seconds before exchanging legs.

Daniel Fishel/Thrillist

Hip flexors: Standing hip flexor stretch

Your hip flexors, the muscles running along the front of your hips, are notorious for shortening and freezing when you go all day sitting. (Again with the sitting!) If you have a desk job, it's especially imperative to require some investment to release them up to help prevent the uneven features that can lead to back pain.

Stand tall, your feet generally hip-separation apart, your knees somewhat bent.

- Take a wide step forward with your right foot, the two feet positively planted on the ground.
- Keeping your chest and middle tall, twist the two knees marginally and sink your hips an inch or two, as though entering a "baby lunge."
- From this position, fold your hips under and press them forward until you feel a stretch through the front of your left hip. Hold for 20 to 30 seconds before exchanging sides.
- Sit on a mat; your knees bowed, feet level on the floor. Position the center of your strap under your right foot, then hold the parts of the strap in each hand.
- Lie back on the mat, then lift your right foot, squeezing it against the strap. Broaden your right leg completely.

- Draw your right leg up and toward your body, keeping your knee straight. Use your hands to pull the strap gently and stretch out the stretch. At the point when you feel a decent stretch, hold the position for 20 to 30 seconds before exchanging sides.

Daniel Fishel/Thrillist

Calves: Wall-helped calf stretch

Last, however absolutely not the least, is the much-required calf stretch. Your calves get a beating, what with conveying your full body weight around throughout the day, so feel free to allow them a moment of adoration, - it's genuinely the least you can do to keep them upbeat and sound.

- Stand facing a wall, your feet hip-distance apart. Press your palms into the divider at chest height, at that point lunge your right foot in reverse, planting your foot on the ground, bowing your front knee varying, yet keeping your back knee straight.
- With your middle straight, lean forward into the divider, stretching the rear of your right calf. At the point when you feel a decent stretch, hold for 20 to 30 seconds before exchanging sides.

At-home exercises to loosen up your hip flexors

There are only a few things more painful than hip flexors that quit working how they should. Running from a dull ache to stabbing pains in the pelvis or crotch region, issues with hip flexors can come from abuse, underuse, improper use, and an absence of good stretching propensities. Luckily, there are four at-home exercises that are intended to loosen up these muscles and offer relief from pain or inconvenience.

One Knee Up

Bow on the floor on one knee with the other foot planted on the floor. With your pelvis tucked under your hips, gently push your body forward as you keep your back straight. When you start to feel the stretch in your upper thigh, quit pushing forward and instead hold the stretch for 30 seconds. You may find that the more you hold the stretch, the simpler it becomes. Gently inch forward again until you feel the stretch in your upper thigh. Switch legs. Repeat multiple times per leg. Try not to hold this stretch for longer than 30-second interims, as it won't improve your adaptability and may bring about an injury.

All Fours

Bind one lower leg to a seat or post with opposition tubing. On your hands and knees, gradually bring the knee of the attached lower leg to your chest. Hold for 5 seconds and gradually return it to the beginning position. You should feel resistance in the two bearings as your hip flexor attempts to move your hip to and fro. Complete two sets of 10 repetitions on every leg.

Seated Hip Flexor Stretch

This is a perfect exercise to do while sitting in an office seat. Change the seat stature so when your feet are planted on the floor, your leg forms a 90-degree angle at your knee. With one foot on the floor, raise the other leg, so it is straight before you, parallel to the floor. Keeping it straight, raise it until your leg is waist-high, at that point lower it, so it is parallel to the floor. Repeat two sets of 10 repetitions on each leg.

Marching Stretch

Standing upright and tall, carry one leg up as hidden from plain view as conceivable just as if you are walking straight up. Hold it there for 5 seconds then, return it to the beginning position. Repeat with the other leg. If you can't adjust viably on one foot, an equivalent exercise should be possible with your back near a wall. Make certain to remain as straight as possible while stretching and exchanging legs.

Probably the ideal approaches to avoid hip flexor pain is to abstain from remaining seated for a long time. The individuals who are physically active or who take occasional breaks from seated work are less inclined to have pain after some time. Regardless of whether you have a normal exercise schedule, guaranteeing your core muscles are solid and can balance out your hips and will significantly influence your degree of pain in your hips.

www.ingramcontent.com/pod-product-compliance
Lightning Source LLC
Chambersburg PA
CBHW070714250726
48662CB00001B/418